PANDE
BLUNDER

Fauci and Public Health
Blocked Early Home COVID Treatment

JOEL S. HIRSCHHORN

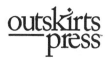

Outskirts Press, Inc.
http://www.outskirtspress.com

ISBN: 978-1-9772-3822-1

Library of Congress Control Number: 2021900097

PRINTED IN THE UNITED STATES OF AMERICA

Preface

This book is for truth-seekers seriously searching for information that can alleviate their anxiety and stress, and possibly their COVID-19 infection. It unravels what the pandemic blunder is, what has caused it, how it impacts your life, and most importantly, how you can survive it and escape its many negative impacts on American lives in this crisis environment.

It presents different types of information regarding health and health care. It should be used to supplement and not replace the advice of your doctor or some other trained health professional, particularly with regard to diagnosing health issues and the use of medicines and supplements. All efforts have been made to assure the accuracy of the information presented at the time of writing and publishing this book; however, the topics covered are very much under scrutiny in the current pandemic. On a daily basis there is a very large number of new articles in medical journals, magazines, and newspapers, as well as on numerous websites. The main goal has been to present credible examples rather than an exhaustive description of a number of topics covered. The publisher and author disclaim liability for any medical outcomes that may occur as a result of using any of the information presented in this book. The author has no financial interest in any of the medicines or supplements discussed in this book. And he does not endorse any specific company or sources or suppliers of medicines, therapeutics, or supplements that are mentioned in this book.

Another important point is that no attempt has been made to cover in any detail the enormous number of negative articles, studies, reports, and news accounts criticizing the many facets of early home/outpatient treatment for COVID infection. This book presents the positive case and the failures of government agencies and the public health system. Roughly, 90 percent or much more of all pandemic coverage either ignores the positive case or criticizes it.

Moreover, considering how rapidly all aspects of the pandemic are moving, there will undoubtedly be considerable new information for quite a while after publication of this book. But one thing will not change: the big pandemic blunder, cause of massive, widespread pain, suffering, and death.

Dr. Hirschhorn is a member of the Association of American Physicians and Surgeons, and America's Frontline Doctors, both extremely active in promoting early home covid treatment.

Foreword

The mismanagement of the Covid-19 pandemic is akin to mass murder, and genocide of the elderly and infirm. The root cause of this crime against humanity is the denial of man's divine origin.

Despite a plethora of scientific data, lifesaving information and access to vital medications is being suppressed from the majority of the human race. This led to the tragic and preventable deaths of over two million people worldwide. The perpetrators of this historically heinous crime are motivated by the desire for power and control over the human race. These modern day slave-masters believe that they are ubermensch (superhuman) with the right to decide who should live or die.

In the last year, I have personally witnessed the tragic and preventable deaths of hundreds of people from Covid-19. Despite a samsonian effort to advocate for effective, safe, and affordable prehospital treatments, my colleagues and I have been threatened and censored.

It is my supposition that this suppression of lifesaving information and medication is mass murder. This crime against humanity has been willfully perpetrated by a group of sociopathic despots that possess a delusional "G-d complex" and perceive themselves as superhumans with the right to enslave others. It is my strong hope and prayer that they will be brought to justice in both the earthly and heavenly courts.

Vladimir Zev Zelenko, M.D.

Table of Contents

Part 1

—⁓—

Understanding the Big Pandemic Blunder

1.1 How big a mistake?

The fundamental premise of this book is that a huge mistake has been made in the way the government at all levels has managed the COVID-19 pandemic. "Huge" and "mistake" don't tell the whole story. A mistake implies an action that is accidental or unintentional. Maybe even one that can be corrected. "Huge" is also inadequate when it comes to the world of medicine and public health.

An astronomical blunder is a more accurate way of describing what has happened in this pandemic. To be clear, what this book is about is an intentional action with enormous, adverse, irreversible consequences and health impacts for large numbers of people. When it comes to life or death, we enter the world of homicide. There are deliberate actions that directly impair human health and, in the extreme, cause avoidable, preventable death. To be clearer, for this pandemic, the correct notion is criminally negligent homicide resulting from intentional actions by myriad government officials.

The pandemic big blunder defined in this book results from an ineffective and incompetent large public health system. There are fifty-six state and territorial public health agencies and nearly 3,000 local agencies. They have always been responsible for dealing with emergencies and urgent health threats as well as preventing disease. The US has about 500,000 public health workers. There are about thirty-two US schools of public health that graduate about 16,000 individuals yearly, and graduate programs producing 800 people with a master of public health, health administration, or health educator degree. Some states require certain credentials for public health officials such as a medical license or specialized training in preventive medicine or public health. What has shaped the pandemic blunder across the whole public health system are the federal agencies, namely the National Institutes of Health, the Centers for Disease Control and Prevention, and the Food and Drug Administration.

Government officials have been supported by a host of allies, principally reporters and commentators in the leftist media, wrong-headed academics, medical societies, medical journals, drug companies, and many leftists in the political world. Inevitably, we must address the causes of the intentional actions and behaviors. Later, both outright corruption and greed will be explored to help answer the inevitable, logical question: How could such a horrendous blunder happen and persist for so long? Is it just a bureaucratic blunder or is it closer to evil intent? If you have any friend or relative who has suffered or died in this pandemic, then you will, by the end of this book, be inclined to think more in terms of evil than incompetence or even merely greed.

As we all cannot help but notice the daily increasing numbers of COVID cases and deaths breathlessly reported by the press, it takes some discipline to mindfully stay in touch with the concept of a disastrous blunder. That blunder explains the constantly rising number of COVID hospitalizations and deaths. Far from the public view is a lot of very positive information and data that can and should cause considerable optimism about having really good early home/outpatient treatment for COVID. This will be explored in detail at a later point. But be assured that it is extremely important to differentiate between treatment given to hospitalized patients versus treatment given to keep people from needing to go to a hospital emergency room.

Understand that all this positive "news" is intentionally kept from public view because it does not fit the negative narrative pushed aggressively by the leftist media in defense of the government officials and agencies responsible for withholding what can safely address your COVID infection at home, which is of critical importance for people with serious underlying health problems and an advanced age.

This brings us to the important strategy tied closely to the big blunder subject of this book, namely maintaining fear in people. The more you stay in a fear mindset, the more difficult it will be to openly inhale the many truths offered in this book and rebel against the medical and public health system that has failed you. Pandemic fear is the weapon used to control the population.

Psychiatrist Mark McDonald has defined a delusional psychosis produced by the pandemic. He noted that fear is the "driving force of the coronavirus pandemic and the hysteria" around it. "Fear has become a new virtue. Never before in the history of this country have we told people that fear is good," or to "settle into" those fears and allow them "to control and constrain your life," said the doctor. Moreover, the pandemic "hysteria" has reached the stage of "going beyond fear, going beyond the crazy itself, to what I would call group control," he said. By keeping a lot of positive information from people, those in power have intentionally fed fear hysteria and anxiety.

Another aspect of this fear society is that ordinary people are increasingly being asked by government to "rat" on others who are not complying with contagion controls. In other words, the US is rapidly using its own citizens as a de facto police force. This seems very similar to communist China, which deliberately created a society where neighbor informs on neighbor, family informs on family. This is pandemic madness.

One final, very important point is this: If the big blunder or pandemic malpractice thesis of this book is correct—which by the end of this book you will likely agree with—then the whole notion that the COVID infection has created a genuine crisis should be seen more as propaganda than a medical reality. There is just as much a disinformation pandemic than a viral one. This "false" pandemic has ruined the American economy and destabilized the society. If the big blunder is widely understood, then the COVID pandemic can end through the use of a proven early home/outpatient treatment and cure. Is this a "magic wand"? A lot of data says it is.

For example, in November 2020, Dr. Vladimir Zelenko, a pioneer in developing and using home/outpatient treatments, was correct when he said that they could have saved over 200,000 lives, when there were nearly 280,000 reported American COVID deaths. A savings of about 70 percent is consistent with results in a number of foreign nations, which will be examined in detail later. If the nation still had a constitutionally protected free and independent press, then there would be screaming headlines how over 200,000 American lives could have been saved with a low-cost, safe home COVID treatment. But the public has been kept away from such truth by a corrupt leftist press.

1.2 The history of medicine message

You don't have to be a physician to appreciate that whenever any illness or disease is discovered or confronted, the prudent approach is to take action to offset the negative health impacts as quickly as possible. This is what patients want and expect. This is what physicians are morally and professionally expected to do. The moral imperative for physicians of "first do no harm" clearly implies not to wait, but rather to take the earliest possible action to fully examine, diagnose, and treat whatever illness or disease a patient has symptoms for. We go to doctors to get early action. If we ignore our own symptoms, then we have to shoulder the blame.

But we have every right to believe that the medical, health care, and public health systems will do everything possible to take early action to not only address our symptoms expeditiously but also to prevent a worsening of whatever illness or disease afflicts us. If they do not, it is malpractice. We should expect that a physician can accurately address our unhealthy situation by telling us what to do about our lifestyle or diet, taking readily available off-the-shelf medicines or supplements, and also perhaps by prescribing regulated medicines.

We surely expect the medical system to do everything possible to keep us out of the hospital. Becoming a hospital patient is rightfully seen as a last resort, both unpleasant, stressful, likely painful, potentially unsafe, and terribly expensive, even with health insurance. With COVID contagion controls in hospitals, moreover, patients will be isolated from their loved ones, friends, and relatives.

In the context of his treating COVID patients, Dr. Jean-Jacques Rajter said, "You look at early interventions for other diseases, we're very aware that the earlier we intervene the better the outcomes are. So, we know that if we were to use [treatment on] our patients early on, we could decrease the likelihood of having people hospitalized and decrease the burden on the hospital systems. [Treatment] could decrease the economic impact on the economy because people could go back to their normal lives."

The incredulous, almost unbelievable blunder that this book is all about, however, is contrary to all these traditional concepts and responsibilities. Which is why many people may resist believing what is unraveled in this book. Reasonable people will ask:

How can we believe that our entire medical and public health system, facing a most historic and seemingly lethal pandemic, failed us in such a profound way?

How could our government not protect our lives by standing in the way of taking the earliest possible action to address the potential devastating pandemic impacts?

But that is exactly what has happened and what will be explored as we progress here. It turns out that there are well-documented blocks that have been imposed by two federal agencies.

When it comes to early medical action, it is important to recognize that some medications are only effective at an early stage. There are different reasons for this. A major reason is that illnesses and diseases often progress through different phases. What works in the early phase may not work in later phases. This is the case for the coronavirus; it progresses from viral replication to florid pneumonia and lastly to multi-organ attack. The trick is to stop it dead in its tracks at the viral replication phase, which is what pillar one is all about. (See next section.)

An example of a commercial medicine that only works in the initial phase is Tamiflu. Tamiflu is used to treat flu symptoms caused by influenza virus in people who have had symptoms for less than two days. Another example is the dangerous sepsis infection, for which it is imperative to have early treatment to avoid death. Sepsis occurs when an extreme immune system response triggers widespread inflammation throughout the body. This resembles somewhat a later stage of COVID infection.

As will be detailed later, a number of proven protocols for COVID are only effective within the first four to seven days of onset of the infection.

1.3 The four pillars of pandemic management

Facing up to the hard-to-believe blunder theme of this book is made difficult because of the many pandemic-related distractions. It may sound a little too much like a conspiracy, but the truth is that all the entities with power and influence deliberately keep the public focused on many negative and, to a lesser degree, positive distractions.

To understand all this, it is imperative to understand the four basic pillars of pandemic management. Dr. Peter McCullough has pioneered this paradigm (though the order of pillars one and two are reversed in this book to emphasize the importance of pillar one); he is vice chair of Internal Medicine at Baylor University Medical Center and a professor of medicine at Texas A&M College of Medicine.

The first pillar, in terms of timing and importance, is early home/outpatient treatment to keep you healthy and out of the hospital once you either have some clear symptoms of COVID—which government agencies and many other groups do a good job telling you about—or you have taken a COVID test and gotten a positive result.

Dr. McCullough has said: "I can't think of a single viral infection where the best advice is to wait two weeks before we start treatment in the hospital. That is the current NIH recommendations. Americans are appalled by this. We always treat serious viral infections with multiple drugs up front, early. These are principles of treatment."

The most important thing to understand about this first pillar is that it has not been widely used because the federal government has not endorsed, supported, or promoted it. To the contrary it has blocked its use mainly through official guidance from the National Institutes of Health that provides for no early home/outpatient COVID treatment.

Two physician organizations with excellent websites have been at the forefront of bringing attention to and providing useful support for this first pillar:

America's Frontline Doctors
American Association for Physicians and Surgeons

Doctors are prevented by government actions in using early home/ outpatient treatment, and their traditional medical freedom to do what they think best for their patients is destroyed. That is exactly the case now.

The second pillar, which at first might seem as timely as the first pillar, is contagion or infection control. This is what has preoccupied the entire pandemic management and response system. Here are all the actions designed in theory to curb the spread of the coronavirus in all parts of society, both public and private. Perhaps the biggest pandemic lie is that contagion controls are based on good, reliable science. To a great degree this is sheer nonsense. The word science is simply used to justify authoritarian actions by all levels of government. Use of pillar one options is truly based on sound science.

This arena of contagion control has become the major distraction from thinking about and demanding first pillar options.

All your thoughts, emotions, and behaviors are now linked to wearing masks, social distancing, washing hands, not shaking hands, using hand sanitizer, keeping children out of school, avoiding outdoor crowds, and, most contentious, putting up with lockdowns that prevent you from visiting stores, restaurants, and gyms, and possibly from going to work, operating a small business, seeing movies, and going to sporting events of any type.

The wearing of masks, in particular, has been highly controversial. Considerable science says masks have limited benefits for the wearer and others around the wearer. This is what everyone must understand. There is nothing magical about any kind of mask that ordinary people wear. Science tells us that a mask might only protect some bigger particles from being inhaled or spread around, but not very, very small virus particles. Moreover, too many people don't wear masks and simple fabric coverings correctly, meaning no tight fit. And people usually cannot stop touching it, which means that any virus in or on the mask gets transferred into your nose or mouth.

One study that received considerable attention was a Danish mask study involving nearly 5,000 people that took place in the spring and early summer of 2020. The big finding was that there were few statistical differences in infection rates between a group that wore masks and a group that didn't. The rational approach is to wear a mask in certain situations, especially inside places with lots of people and outside in crowds. Note that this study had a hard time getting published because of a widespread bias in favor of masks.

Besides supposedly curbing the spread of the infection, these contagion controls mostly run up against individual and constitutionally protected freedoms. They disrupt our normal social and economic lives. In fact, these contagion control measures and particularly lockdowns cause a host of negative health impacts. People are increasingly suffering because of social isolation and stresses. They are not taking ordinary care for all kinds of non-pandemic health problems as they fear going to doctors and hospitals. Most studies have found that the negatives of lockdowns are equal or greater than the negative impacts of COVID itself. Lives are being devastated and lost because of the array of lockdown contagion controls being used. The health and economic costs do not justify the benefits.

In September 2020, Donald Luskin in the *Wall Street Journal* reached these conclusions: "Lockdowns correlated with a greater spread of the virus. States with longer, stricter lockdowns also had larger COVID outbreaks. The five places with the harshest lockdowns—the District of Columbia, New York, Michigan, New Jersey, and Massachusetts—had the heaviest caseloads. ...[T]here's no escaping the evidence that, at minimum, heavy lockdowns were no more effective than light ones, and that opening up a lot was no more harmful than opening up a little. So, where's the science that would justify the heavy lockdowns many public health officials are still demanding?"

The negative view of lockdowns is not limited to millions of harmed Americans. A November 2020 UNICEF report spoke of a "shadow pandemic of violence against women and children, with vital services to these vulnerable groups being among the most commonly disrupted." And the World Health Organization said in October 2020 that lockdowns should not be "the primary means of control of this virus," noting a lockdown consequence too frequently overlooked this year: "making poor people an awful lot poorer."

The Great Barrington Declaration, created in October 2020 by two distinguished physicians and a senior epidemiologist, now has well over 700,000 signers. It took a strong position on contagion controls, especially lockdowns. Here are some excerpts.

"Current lockdown policies are producing devastating effects on short- and long-term public health. The results (to name a few) include lower childhood vaccination rates, worsening cardiovascular disease outcomes, fewer cancer screenings, and deteriorating mental health—leading to greater excess mortality in years to come, with the working class and younger members of society carrying the heaviest burden. Keeping students out of school is a grave injustice. …Keeping these measures in place until a vaccine is available will cause irreparable damage, with the underprivileged disproportionately harmed. … allow those who are at minimal risk of death to live their lives normally to build up immunity to the virus through natural infection, while better protecting those who are at highest risk. We call this Focused Protection. …Those who are not vulnerable should immediately be allowed to resume life as normal."

In his December 2020 senate testimony, the distinguished Dr. Ramin Oskoui, who has had extensive COVID experience, said that "lockdowns are inappropriate because they do not make scientific or economic sense." He also cited data that indicated hard quarantines, masks, and social distancing are ineffective.

Where's the science? That is the point about contagion controls overall. It is mainly in the delusional minds of their tyrannical proponents.

Dealing with all of these contagion controls defines daily distractions from what should be a priority, namely discovering how you can get effective, early home/outpatient treatment for COVID. But here is the even worse truth. It should be clear after so many months of the government putting so much emphasis on contagion controls that they have not worked very well. If you keep all your attention on these controls, then you have fallen victim to a complex combination of organized propaganda and information suppression. Maybe you do not become a victim of the virus, but you have been made a different kind of victim.

No matter how much effort you put into faithfully obeying what the government tells you to do, you remain at risk of catching the virus anyway. This is the ugly truth for not only Americans but for many people in countries where strong contagion controls have been used, such as in Italy, but where nevertheless there have been ever rising hospitalizations and deaths. Compliance with contagion controls plus distraction do not guarantee that you will escape catching the virus, though you might be asymptomatic but still be contagious. But overall, this is so much worse than having the option to use the first pillar: early home/outpatient treatment within a few days of symptoms or a positive test.

To summarize, you probably will appreciate that the nation's emphasis on contagion control has resulted in these negative impacts:

- The national economy has been wrecked; and the global economy also.
- The lives of millions of Americans have been savaged. Pandemic fatigue is an all too real medical condition that has created mental health problems for many.
- Those with the lowest levels of personal wealth have been especially devastated.
- Untold number of small businesses have been brutalized; many will never come back to life. This has contributed greatly to high unemployment.

- Children have been robbed of a good education because of extensive school closings and the use of ineffective remote learning. Many have also suffered various bad health impacts. All this despite there being no rational scientific basis for the closings, which was first revealed in a study in April 2020. Data available for a long time showed that children do not get serious COVID illness, nor do they transmit significantly to adults.

To add insult to injury is what has been all too frequently revealed in the news, namely a large number of public officials who have blatantly violated their own government contagion controls, mostly mayors and governors.

One more final, important point about contagion controls is that they make the most sense when a bad virus is greatly limited to a tight geographical region like a city or island nation. But once a highly contagious virus is out in the real world, over a large area, contagion controls are not likely to work effectively enough to justify all the pain and dislocation they cause. Sadly, American politicians hungry for power do not seem to have learned this lesson.

To show this reality about where contagion controls can work, consider the extremely low COVID death rates for these island nations: New Zealand – 5; Australia – 35; Japan – 17; and Cuba – 12, compared to over 800 for the US Cuba, however, has also used the home/outpatient treatment to be detailed at a later point.

Controlling people coming into a nation is critical. To be clear, President Trump did the correct thing when he cut travel from China and Europe. But the virus had already spread from China into much

14

of the world in earlier times. Research has shown, for example, that the virus had entered the US in mid-December 2019 and in Italy as early as September 2019, which is consistent with the devastation in Italy (which has a higher COVID death rate than the US) despite vigorous use of contagion controls.

Finally, it must be emphasized that contagion controls have not been based on rigorous randomized controlled trials, to be discussed later, so often cited by Fauci as holding back use of hydroxychloroquine (HCQ).

The third pillar is treatment in a hospital. Clearly, enormous attention has been given to the incredible dedication, sacrifice, and performance of all those providing hospital care for patients with COVID. And there has been endless information of real or potential shortages of hospital capacity for caring for COVID patients. The public is supposed to be terribly frightened that should they catch the virus, they may not be able to find hospital treatment. Once in a hospital you have to hope that they will employ the best actions and medicines. Indeed, these have changed and improved in recent months in a major way. But still, about 25 percent of COVID deaths happen in hospitals.

The fourth pillar is the use of vaccines, which has been given increasing attention as the salvation for ending the pandemic. This is somewhat illusory and also part of the vast propaganda and suppression machine. It also contributes yet another distraction from demanding access to the first pillar. In fact, it is logical to see that the first pillar is a direct competitor to the fourth pillar. If the public was both more aware of effective, safe, and low-cost early home/outpatient treatment and could easily access it, then it would make perfect sense to be less interested in taking a vaccine. This is especially the case now because the government and big drug companies have rushed through the clinical trials and regulatory approvals.

Most surveys in 2020 showed that about 50 percent of Americans were not inclined to get one of the approved vaccines. This may get worse as more attention is given to unpleasant side effects from taking the vaccine. One reason for public apathy about COVID vaccines is what Fauci said in November 2020. "Obviously, with a 90-plus percent effective vaccine, you could feel much more confident. But I would recommend to people to not abandon all public health measures just because you have been vaccinated, because even though, for the general population, it might be 90 to 95 percent effective, you don't necessarily know, for you, how effective it is." In other words, keep obeying all the government dictates for contagion control, such as wearing masks.

Impartial doctors and others have raised serious concerns about the safety and effectiveness of this stream of Operation Warp Speed vaccines. Thus, it is correct to see COVID vaccines as a major distraction from public interest in and demand for the pillar one home/outpatient treatment. If public demand for pillar one treatment could be increased, then surely public interest in pillar four vaccines would decline. The simple reason is that both could be seen as cures for the virus.

Which one could be seen as safer? This is a key but difficult question because for probably a long time the safety of coronavirus vaccines will not be fully understood for different groups of people. The main reason for this uncertainty is the lack of detailed data on exactly what groups of people have been tested for all the vaccines and whether the efficacy and safety were always high, in particular, whether elderly people and children had been adequately tested in the trials. Fauci has advocated children taking the vaccine, even though considerable data have shown that children do not get serious cases of COVID infection. There are also many questions regarding whether getting a vaccine will give people real immunity and for how long. One smart view is that immunity confers protection from severity of illness if reinfected, not that you can't be reinfected.

The rational mindset for Americans is to personally decide whether taking a serious look into how to get early home/outpatient COVID treatment is a wise alternative to automatically getting the vaccine because of what public health officials say.

1.4 Pillars two, three, and four against pillar one

This is a lopsided battle. Let us try to explain the common denominator among the three that are best considered as inferior to the first pillar. It may sound simplistic, but it comes down to one person: Dr. Anthony Fauci, a subject that will be delved into in detail at a later point.

For now, the key fact is that Fauci is the epitome of the bureaucratic establishment. He has served as the director of the National Institute of Allergy and Infectious Diseases (NIAID) since 1984. It is probably impossible to find any other state, local, or federal official who has been in such a high-level position for nearly four decades. An interesting fact is that Fauci is the highest paid employee in the federal government, making more money than the president, well over $400,000 annually.

Fauci is a major culprit of using the pandemic to foster a terribly

17

politicized and polarized society, as well as degrading respect for science and scientists. Tucker Carlson got it right when he said in November 2020 that Fauci had been revealed as a "power-mad incompetent."

Establishment entities protect their turfs and self-interests and have sacrificed the well-being and lives of most Americans in this pandemic. The government is not just the enemy of the people, mind you, but an enemy of a number of other older, prestigious groups. The most important of these is the mainstream media that both spreads propaganda against pillar one options and suppresses a multitude of truths in favor of those options. At the same time, the media pushes propaganda in favor of pillars two, three, and four, trying to convince the public that contagion controls and vaccines offer a "solution" for the pandemic. But most people have become frustrated with contagion controls, and surveys in 2020 showed that about 50 percent of Americans were not inclined to get one of the approved vaccines.

Explaining a wide collusion of all the entities refusing to support early home/outpatient treatment for COVID requires seeing a key political reality. Political forces lined up against President Trump, who upon hearing of the earliest successful home treatments for COVID from doctors went public with support for using hydroxychloroquine (HCQ). In mid-May 2020, he announced he started taking HCQ; this was about two months after several doctors went public with their successful use of HCQ for COVID treatment. Trump took it as a prophylactic against getting COVID. However, he apparently did not take weekly doses, which would be the correct medical approach, so he eventually got the COVID infection.

Add in the most powerful person in the federal government, Dr.

Anthony Fauci, a globalist leftist with strong ties to big pharmaceutical companies. More than anyone else, he got the National Institutes of Health and the Food and Drug Administration to take formal positions against home treatment and use of HCQ. Include the leftist mainstream media waging endless war against Trump. Mix in the medical and public health establishments, including major medical societies that backed the government positions.

The media attack against HCQ was propelled initially by two medical research articles published in two of the most prestigious medical journals. The leftist mainstream media jumped on the negative findings for HCQ. In what has amounted to a remarkable historic event, both articles were retracted soon after a number of people were able to correctly explain that both papers were bogus at best, and possibly intentionally fraudulent. The situation for *The Lancet* and *The New England Journal of Medicine* has been widely seen as a failure of the peer review process used by journals. Both withdrawn articles were accepted very quickly, while many others with positive findings on HCQ could not get accepted.

Those two articles, before their retraction, created a global storm against the use of HCQ. For example, *USA Today* screamed, "Coronavirus patients who took HCQ had higher risk of death, study shows." The World Health Organization ordered nations to stop using HCQ and suspended trials being held in hundreds of hospitals across the world. And France, Italy, and Belgium banned HCQ for COVID-19 trials. Such is the power of negative published studies that feed an anti-HCQ narrative. This is still going on as new published articles in medical journals give negative findings on HCQ that have no merit or applicability to early home/outpatient use.

An interesting example of how broad the disinterest in pillar one is the major media exposure given to successful author Alex Berenson. He has devoted himself to finding and articulating problems with contagion control measures, all well and good. But he has ignored the inattention to the pillar one option and, therefore, has not recognized the big pandemic blunder.

1.5 The weaponization of data

We all are inundated daily with pandemic data. The key issue is whether you can trust the data and how it is being interpreted by government authorities and the media. The data tell us how effective or ineffective contagion controls are.

First consider the number of cases hyped every day by the media. If you trust the various testing protocols, then this tells you how many people have tested positive for the virus. The positivity rate is that percentage of all the tests that produced a positive test result. The lower that number, the better the pandemic situation is. In many countries and the US, that rate is 10 percent or more. Clearly, the more testing done, the more cases will be revealed.

Many health and other professionals have raised concerns about whether case numbers which always are on the rise accurately assess the spread of the virus and the danger to the public. The rising number of cases is used to continue using abusive and intrusive contagion controls. Some tests, however, produce false positives. Some measure extremely low levels of virus that pose no harm or threat. And a very high number of cases, some say about 40 percent, represent asymptomatic conditions where virus loads in the body may be too low to cause virus spreading or show up in a test.

In the most common PCR (polymerase chain reaction) test, a major problem is the cycle count, that is, how many multiple cycles of amplification are used to yield a detectable amount of RNA. It is supposed to determine how much virus the person harbors. But many labs use as high as forty cycles, which can pick up fragments of the coronavirus but not enough for the person to be sick or contagious. This causes many PCR tests to yield false positive results. Most experts think that about twenty cycles are optimal to reveal genuine COVID illness. If there is some kind of pressure to find increased numbers of cases, then labs might run tests to get higher numbers of infection. This can easily result in misleading information on the pandemic, because so many positive tests do not really indicate a serious COVID infection or that a person can spread the disease.

On the issue of false positive test data, there are serious impacts not just for individuals who pursue medical and possibly hospital care. On a larger level, the political and media attention to new waves of the coronavirus may be a scam. In an *American Thinker*, December 2020 article, Dr. Mike Yeadon, former chief scientific officer and V.P., and allergy and respiratory research head with Pfizer Global R&D, argues that false positive results from inherently unreliable COVID tests are being used to manufacture a "second wave" based on "new cases." He "warned that if half of tests for COVID-19 are false positives. ...We are basing a government policy, an economic policy, a civil liberties policy ... on what may well be completely erroneous data on this coronavirus."

The other issue with testing is getting a false negative, meaning you have an infection and may be contagious. A negative test may be irrelevant if a person becomes exposed significantly to the virus after the test. What is a person to do? Take test after test? Megan McArdle in the *Washington Post* made this wise comment about testing: "At the individual level it is borderline useless." In other words, testing all too easily creates a false feeling of safety and security.

In November 2020, Elon Musk made headlines when he went public about his experience with rapid COVID testing. "Something extremely bogus is going on. Two tests came back negative, two came back positive. Same machine, same test, same nurse," he said.

Most people get a polymerase chain reaction (PCR) test. These are known to have a false negative rate of up to 30 percent. Musk had faster antigen tests, which are even less accurate.

False negative PCR test results are a big problem. A study published in the *Annals of Internal Medicine*, for example, found that there is a 100 percent chance of a negative test on the day of exposure, 38 percent after five days, around the time symptoms begin, and 20 percent three days later. Dr. Lauren Kucirka observed, "There's never a time that you can rely on [the test] 100 percent" to know whether you are really negative. This may explain why so many COVID victims end up in hospital after the infection proceeds to advanced stages and severe symptoms.

One thing is very true. Many companies are making a ton of money selling tests. And millions of Americans go through hell trying to get tested.

As to case numbers, they can and should include the numbers for recovered patients and deaths. Worldwide about 97 percent of closed cases are in the recovered or discharged category, and about 3 percent are deaths. Deaths per million population (not the total number of cases or deaths) is the proper way of seeing how lethal the coronavirus is in a specific nation, state, or locality. The death rate is very high for a number of countries, not just the US, typically over 700 or 800 per million people. Rates for states vary greatly, well over 1,500 for New York, New Jersey, and Massachusetts, and a number of states with less than 500 per million, including, for example, Virginia, Washington, Oregon, Utah, Maine, Alaska, and Vermont.

It helps to remember that less than 1 percent of the US population accounts for over 90 percent of all the deaths, and most of these occur in people over age seventy, mostly over age eighty, with at least two and a half to three comorbidities, according to the CDC. About 40 percent of deaths have occurred in nursing and assisted living facilities.

You may ask: Why is there so much variation in pandemic statistics? There are three main answers: use and effectiveness of contagion controls and, as will be delved into later, whether some nations have used pillar one options. Some states that have used less coercive contagion controls have done just as well as others pursuing more intrusive actions. But the most concerning problem with varying death rates is that many governments (both states and foreign nations) use extremely different rationales for defining a death as due to the coronavirus. There have been many situations revealing a determination to count deaths as COVID, even though that is ludicrous all too often. One reason for this is that the Medicare program provides hospitals with a 20 percent bonus for COVID patients.

An old piece of medical wisdom for prostate cancer is that most men will die with prostate cancer but not from it. The same appears true for the COVID situation. Those with COVID symptoms or a positive test result (even after death) are often categorized as COVID deaths, even for people committing suicide, dying in an accident, or dying from a well-established, serious medical condition. The ugly truth though is that high case numbers work wonderfully to assist authoritarian governments to use coercive contagion controls.

Second, numbers on hospitalization rates are of considerable importance. The failure of contagion controls gets translated into hospitalization numbers, which increase greatly with a patient's age, especially those who are over seventy and eighty years old. Whether individual hospitals, however, are overloaded and incapable of taking in new COVID patients is a very different matter. The leftist media all too often spreads fear about hospital capacity shortages.

Two of the major websites used to get pandemic data—a Johns Hopkins site and the worldometers site—do not give hospitalization rates. The COVID tracking website presents national data for the US Typical numbers in recent times reveal that over 90,000 Americans are in hospital with COVID infection, and somewhat fewer than 20,000 are in ICU units. Becker's hospital review site presents state data on hospital COVID patients, which vary greatly.

In November 2020, the CDC provided these figures: 2.4 million hospitalizations, 44.8 million symptomatic illnesses, and 52.9 million total infections may have occurred in the US population from February 27–September 30, 2020. These indicate that a 4.5 percent hospitalization has occurred.

Worth noting is a Johns Hopkins study that looked very closely at normal versus COVID deaths. It raised the issue of whether a drop in normally expected deaths is offset by legitimate COVID deaths. Here is what was observed:

"The effect of COVID-19 on deaths in the U.S. is considered problematic only when it increases the total number of deaths or the true death burden by a significant amount in addition to the expected deaths by other causes. Since the crude number of total deaths by all causes before and after COVID-19 has stayed the same, one can hardly say that COVID-19 deaths are concerning. ... The goal is never to undermine the effects of COVID-19 but to suggest a possible over-exaggeration in death numbers due to the pandemic."

In other words, this analysis strongly suggests that deaths due to heart diseases, respiratory diseases, influenza, and pneumonia, for example, may instead be recategorized as being due to COVID-19. Another possibility is that COVID infection is occurring earlier than death from conventional causes in people with serious comorbidities. But such deaths are not necessarily a direct result of COVID. Many physicians believe that official COVID death numbers are too high and these are used by fearmongers to help political forces control the population.

The CDC has said that only 6 percent of COVID deaths were solely due to COVID (without comorbidities) and that all the rest might have been related to COVID. But that opens the door to concerns that many different rationales are used to justify listing a death as a COVID one. How can the public know that COVID has actually contributed to many deaths, especially for the elderly?

Often, the US has been condemned for having much high numbers of COVID cases and deaths than other first world, industrialized nations such as Germany. But the sad fact is that Americans are unhealthier and have greater comorbidities than people in other such countries. Plus, our health care system is more likely to have perverse effects from financial incentives for hospitalization. Death rates in other countries may be more reliable than those in the US.

The main point worth emphasizing is that pandemic data are used to justify investments and actions by governments in pursuing actions under pillars two, three, and four, but not to rethink their strategies and pursue pillar one options. Also at play are financial benefits for this overall strategy directly to the health care system and, indirectly, to drug companies selling expensive medicines and vaccines, and others selling tests. Finally, the angrier Americans have become about the way the pandemic has damaged their lives, the more that data is used to combat this rational anger and suppress public understanding of the big blunder by the entire public health system.

1.6 The leftist problem

It is indisputable that there is a definite leftist dimension to the big blunder. When it comes to understanding the pandemic blunder, it is prudent to see leftists as religious zealots and terrorists and not scientists. Their weapon is fear. By inducing enough fear among people, personal liberty can be squashed by authoritarian governments in the name of fighting the pandemic.

The attack of the leftists started when President Trump went public early in the pandemic with a very positive view of using the low-cost generic medicine hydroxychloroquine to fight the virus—medicine used for many, many decades to address a number of diseases and for which billions of prescriptions have been given worldwide. The leftist media jumped on this, even though starting in March a number of innovative doctors, especially Dr. Zelenko mentioned earlier, had been using the drug successfully to keep COVID patients healthy and out of the hospital.

Even as more and more solid data were being revealed about pillar one options being successful, this was ignored while at the same time the many negative data on COVID cases, hospitalizations, and deaths were emphasized. All this seemed to be a strategy to make Trump and his handling of the pandemic appear ineffective.

When Trump argued in July 2020 for opening schools, he was strongly criticized by the leftist press. Months later he was proven correct. Fauci begrudgingly admitted, finally, schools should be reopened, but not until November.

One interesting example of this leftist phenomenon was a full US Senate committee hearing in November 2020 with the title "Early Outpatient Treatment: An Essential Part of a COVID-19 Solution." Three outstanding witnesses who advocated pillar one actions testified, including Dr. Peter McCullough and Dr. George Fareed (frontline clinicians with great experience treating COVID patients) and Dr. Harvey Risch, a renowned Yale University professor of epidemiology. The Republican Chairman, Ron Johnson of Wisconsin, and several other Republican members supported what those three witnesses said.

"I'm asking for the government to organize all government agencies that are related to this to assist doctors rapidly with their innovation and their compassionate care of patients with COVID-19 at home," McCullough said.

But all of the Democrat members totally avoided any questions or attention to the early treatment topic of the hearing; they gave all their attention to contagion control and vaccines. The Democrat members had placed one witness for the hearing, an academic physician, and he was no supporter of early treatment and had to admit that he had never treated a COVID patient.

Johnson summed up the ugly reality perfectly. He said it was "unconscionable and inhumane" to do nothing to promote effective home treatments. And he said this: "We should have the right to access this without the interference of bureaucrats in the CDC, NIH, and the FDA. And that is exactly what's happened. I can't get it. Millions of Americans can't access it because of the disinformation, the scaremongering, and the prescription log jam that has been created by bureaucrats. …We can't wait for the vaccine; we have to take action now."

Johnson made another important point. He wondered aloud whether doctors and medical experts were backing another drug, remdesivir, only for hospitalized COVID patients, over hydroxychloroquine because remdesivir sales bring in more money for pharmaceutical companies. "I question the fact that because this cocktail costs about $20 and remdesivir costs $3,000, that maybe there's a little bias, maybe there's a little conflict, maybe there's a little agenda," he said. Later, more will be reported on the remdesivir disgrace.

When it comes to very expensive new drugs like remdesivir, it should be noted that they and many drugs and vaccines were developed with NIH money, resulting in about $100 million annually in royalties. In other words, NIH makes a lot of money from drug companies that it has a close relationship with.

After the hearing, the mainstream leftist media gave no attention to the success of early home/outpatient treatment, and only maintained their focus on how bad the pandemic and its handling by Trump was. In the *Wall Street Journal* Holman Jenkins, Jr. made the sage observation that after the hearing, the press "mostly reverted to the story line that HCQ is a useless drug that Mr. Trump promoted."

Senator Johnson held a second hearing on the same topic in December. Again, Democrats boycotted it. Six impressive physicians from the private sector testified. Senator Rand Paul made the point that there is "too much confidence in government doctors, such as Dr. Fauci."

One might ask: Why hasn't the leftist media condemned the Trump administration for not pursuing pillar one options? The best answer is that it would place Fauci in a very difficult position because more than anyone else he is the cause for the big blunder of ignoring pillar one options. Let there be no doubt. Fauci is a leftist. The mainstream media coverage literally every day is truly amazing. He is always referred to in the most glowing ways as if he is some gift from God. Much more will be provided on Fauci later in this book.

1.7 Guilt does not reverse wrongheaded thinking

A very large number of people and organizations that have been pushing pillars two, three, and four over pillar one should feel guilty of betraying the public. But in truth they do not seem to suffer guilt.

29

There is no indication that the pandemic guilty ones will ever respect an incredible amount of solid medical data showing the safety and efficacy of early home/outpatient treatment. Their stubbornness makes them guilty of literally killing several hundred thousand Americans. Rather than admit that they have backed the wrong measures, they will cling to their positions. To do otherwise would place all the advocates for pillars two, three, and four facing the prospect of accepting responsibility for what will amount to several hundred thousand American deaths, such as the 200,000 figure given by Dr. Zelenko mentioned earlier. They will not accept their deserved guilt for the big pandemic blunder. There is much too much cognitive dissonance at stake.

Unfortunately, public officials are not likely to be prosecuted for criminally negligent homicide for killing so many thousands of Americans who could have been saved from COVID through early home/outpatient treatment. The best case for such prosecution is New York State Governor Andrew Cuomo. Despite very wide publicity about his March 2020 mandate to send over 6,300 elderly COVID victims from hospitals into unprepared nursing homes where so many died, he has never publicly accepted responsibility. Even more have died in New York nursing homes over time.

A White House official said: "His reckless response did not follow CMS and CDC guidelines, devastating the senior population—and no amount of revisionist history can erase Governor Cuomo's grossly incompetent decision."

As of late November 2020, the New York State COVID death rate was nearly 1,800 per million population, over twice the rate for the whole country and nine times greater than that for the whole world.

The rate is greater than any single nation on the planet, with nearly 35,000 deaths, very high compared to all nations.

Despite all this bad news, Governor Cuomo has never publicly accepted responsibility or expressed guilt, showing the unlikeliness that other public officials will ever confess their mistake in not promoting early home/outpatient treatment in this pandemic. No amount of solid data seems to have the power to overcome repressed guilt.

Part 2

—∿—

The Positive Case for Early Home/Outpatient COVID Treatment

2.1 The attack on hydroxychloroquine's effectiveness and safety

NIH officially says in its COVID-19 treatment guidelines that it "does not recommend any specific antiviral or immunomodulatory therapy for the treatment of COVID-19" for non-hospitalized patients. This puts physicians in a terrible position who want to use what works and causes the vast majority of American doctors to avoid using what has been proven safe and effective for those infected by the coronavirus who are still at home. Moreover, over forty state medical and pharmacy licensing boards and governors prohibit doctors from prescribing HCQ and patients from obtaining it. What NIH has done is to set in legal stone a rejection of pillar one early home/outpatient COVID treatment.

Of course, a number of courageous doctors take risks and prescribe HCQ anyway. But they represent a small fraction of all American doctors. Thus, relatively few Americans are getting HCQ, meaning that many end up in hospital, adding to the constantly negative data pushed by the media and signaling a terrible pandemic.

Likewise, the FDA does not give approval for HCQ use for treating the coronavirus. This makes it difficult to get HCQ when there is any sign that it is being prescribed for COVID patients.

All this is a conspiracy of incompetent government and public health officials that, as will be shown, is killing enormous numbers of Americans.

In his essay "How Expert Worship Is Ruining Science," in *The American Mind*, Pasha Kamyshev made this astute observation: "The debate over HCQ has both sides thinking the other is killing people. One side happens to be right. History will not judge those who were wrong on this very kindly." Most of us who have seriously examined the pandemic and you who seriously consider the information presented here know that HCQ is saving lives, and history should strongly condemn all those who have fought its use. But that will come long after enormous numbers of people will die unnecessarily from the COVID infection.

Before getting into details about positive results for the use of HCQ, it is appropriate to address the assault on it by all those against pillar one early home/outpatient treatment. The reason for this attack is that the early and still dominant treatment protocols use HCQ. And as mentioned earlier, the advocacy for HCQ by President Trump motivated the leftist attempt to undermine use of HCQ. The array of attacks has been correctly described as an "assassination" attempt. And not just the killing of HCQ, but also of American lives.

To the extent that there remains a marked under use of the pillar one approach to COVID infection, the many attacks on HCQ have been successful, despite having no medical credibility if all the medical evidence is fairly examined. The big blunder started with myriad attacks on HCQ, despite its approved use by the FDA for some sixty-five years and many millions of prescriptions—and billions worldwide—for its use for a number of diseases, such as malaria and lupus. It is genuinely difficult to understand how such a widely used medicine, available as a very low-cost generic, could be so viciously attacked. There had to be ulterior motives. There were, including attacking Trump, protecting the priority of using pillars two, three, and four rather than pillar one, and making billions of dollars for big drug companies.

Another factor in understanding HCQ attacks is the conflict of interest that many in the medical world have because they stand to profit from the use of expensive medicines and vaccines, as well as regulators in bed with drug companies. Dr. Harvey Risch focused on this in an October 2020 article in the *Washington Examiner* and, in particular, the role of the FDA, which is tightly bound to drug companies. He summed it up this way: "Many or most of the 220,000 deaths in the United States to date could have been prevented by widespread HCQ use that the FDA blocked. It is the FDA that is responsible for these deaths, not the president. It is sheer corrupt hypocrisy, and completely shameful, for past FDA commissioners and for a *New England Journal of Medicine* editor with ties to the FDA to accuse the president of what the FDA itself has done."

Perhaps the best overall analysis of the HCQ issue is the article "Hydroxychloroquine: A Morality Tale" by Norman Doidge, published in the *Tablet Magazine* in August 2020. The provocative subtitle is: "A startling investigation into how a cheap, well-known drug became a political football in the midst of a pandemic." The said that HCQ had cut the death rate in half and that worldwide HCQ might save a million lives before the pandemic was tamed.

Also noted was that "early in the coronavirus pandemic, a survey of the world's frontline physicians showed hydroxychloroquine to be the drug they considered the most effective at treating COVID-19 patients. That was in early April, shortly after a French study showed it was safe and effective in lowering the virus count, at times in combination with azithromycin."

The dark side of our current reality was captured by Doidge thusly: "We live in a culture that has uncritically accepted that every domain of life is political, and that even things we think are not political are so, that all human enterprises are merely power struggles, that even the idea of 'truth' is a fantasy, and really a matter of imposing one's view on others. For a while, some held out hope that science remained an exception to this. That scientists would not bring their personal political biases into their science, and they would not be mobbed if what they said was unwelcome to one faction or another. But the sordid 2020 drama of hydroxychloroquine—which saw scientists routinely attacked for critically evaluating evidence and coming to politically inconvenient conclusions—has, for many, killed those hopes."

So, when some people in power talk about following the science, there is much to question about what they mean and what their possible hidden agenda is.

In this regard, Doidge makes another great point: "What is unique about the hydroxychloroquine discussion is that it is a story of 'unwishful thinking'—to coin a term for the perverse hope that some good outcome that most sane people would earnestly desire will never come to pass." To a large degree this turns out to be true, because those fighting to promote the use of HCQ have not succeeded very much against all the forces opposing it, to the detriment of protecting American lives.

All this fits perfectly with the premise of this book, namely that there has been the big pandemic blunder by which people and institutions with power have refused to accept the legitimacy of pillar one; that is, that early home/outpatient treatment really does offer a genuine solution to the COVID pandemic. The cheap, effective, and safe cure is a reality.

Doidge knows what is really going on, when he says "medications and vaccines are competing to Save the World—and for the billions of dollars that will go along with that." The HCQ story really is about powerful forces willing to let untold numbers of people die because they want some entities to make tons of money by pursuing pillars three and four options.

In the article "Hydroxychloroquine and the Crisis of Reality" by Dennis Behreandt in *The New American*, these conclusions about HCQ merit attention. He noted that there have been "far too many deaths of those who died of COVID unnecessarily—including those who did not get HCQ treatments that might have helped them. ...

There are material results that strongly suggest that using hydroxychloroquine is a valid and helpful approach in treating COVID patients. Notwithstanding those results and the actual experiences of doctors and patients with the treatment, much effort has been expended by those aligned with the international 'progressive' apparatus—of which the American Democrat Party and mainstream media are key parts—to construct an alternative paradigm in which, among other things, hydroxychloroquine is both ineffective and dangerous."

As to the safety of HCQ, Dr. Harvey Risch in his October 2020 article made this point about HCQ: "The FDA does not mention that it has no data showing adverse events in outpatient use. In short, among relatively healthy outpatients, HCQ has amassed one of the deepest and most extensive safety records of any drug in history, and the FDA's warning implication of general harm is an outright lie." In his November 2020 testimony at the Senate hearing, he said HCQ "is exceedingly safe." He made this medical point, namely that it had been used for some sixty-five years "without routine screening EKGs, given to adults, children, pregnant women, and nursing mothers, must be safe in the initial viral-replication phase of an illness (COVID) that is similar at that point to colds or flu."

As to the safety of HCQ, the Doidge article mentioned earlier cited work by Dr. Risch. "When its foes speak of frightening side effects, they do so without ever quantifying how common they are. [Risch] found that of 300,000 people with multiple illnesses, who had been tried on the medication combination (HCQ in a cocktail) worldwide, the number of cardiac arrhythmias was 47 per 100,000 and the number of deaths (the key figure) was 9 per 100,000. This was at a time when 10,000 Americans were dying every week from COVID-19."

Doidge went on: "Confirmation bias against HCQ has been so intense, especially among those who don't have experience prescribing it, that the bias-holders simply ignore large studies like Ford (Michigan hospital system) and brush aside the fact that the drug had been safe enough to be a standard of care for decades."

Much detailed data on the safety of HCQ is given in the readily available White Paper on hydroxychloroquine by Dr. Simone Gold on the website of America's Frontline Doctors. There is absolutely no question that HCQ is safe, with the one exception that has occurred in some badly designed studies on hospitalized patients where the dose was extremely high, way above 400 milligrams per day.

Nevertheless, there are many medical journal articles trying to condemn HCQ because of a lack of safety. They are not to be trusted, especially when one recalls that over many billions of HCQ prescriptions have been safely used worldwide.

2.2 Positive protocols and studies

An interesting historic note is how some doctors in China made a most important observation in the first few months of 2020. As recounted by Doidge: "Chinese physicians at the People's Hospital of Wuhan University told their Western counterparts that they got the idea of using HCQ because none of the 178 patients they had admitted for COVID-19 had lupus—a surprise, since lupus is an immune disease, and some thought it might have made these patients especially vulnerable. They wondered why this might be, and whether HCQ, which these patients had been taking for this preexisting condition, might in some way be protecting them against COVID-19." It turns out that they had latched on to the right thing.

The China observation did not go unnoticed. The next historic event was the brilliant work of the renowned French scientist Didier Raoult, who came up with the idea of combining the two older drugs, HCQ and azithromycin, for COVID-19. He found definite benefits for his cocktail when given early in a patient's infection. As reported in April 2020, his study in Marseille, France, involved 1,061 COVID-19 patients, treated for at least three days with the hydroxychloroquine-azithromycin (HCQ-AZ) combination, and a follow-up of at least nine days was investigated. No cardiac toxicity was observed. A good clinical outcome and virological cure were obtained in 973 patients within ten days (91.7%). A poor outcome was observed for forty-six patients (4.3%); ten were transferred to intensive care units; five patients died (0.47%) (74-95 years old); and thirty-one required ten days of hospitalization or more.

The conclusion was: "The HCQ-AZ combination, when started immediately after diagnosis, is a safe and efficient treatment for COVID-19, with a mortality rate of 0.5%, in elderly patients. It avoids worsening and clears virus persistence and contagiosity in most cases." Raoult has suffered incredible attacks in France, which banned the use of HCQ, despite the fact that the death rate in Marseille, where HCQ was used, was much lower than the death rate in the rest of France.

Despite all the impediments, Raoult had treated over 3,700 patients, and the fatality rate was less than 1 percent compared to a death rate in the rest of France of more than 15 percent. This was the June 2020 published conclusion: "Although this is a retrospective analysis, results suggest that early diagnosis, early isolation and early treatment of COVID-19 patients, with at least 3 days of HCQ-AZ lead to a significantly better clinical outcome and a faster viral load reduction than other treatments."

The details of the treatment of 3,737 patients were published: 200 milligrams of oral HCQ three times daily for ten days, and 500 milligrams of oral AZ on day one, followed by 250 milligrams daily for the next four days, respectively. There were no cases of abnormal heart rhythm or sudden death. It should be noted that this key publication by Raoult and his colleagues was in a rather obscure publication, *Travel Medicine and Infectious Disease,* probably because of difficulty getting it published by more prestigious journals with some bias against HCQ.

For more impressive evidence consider the November 2020 Senate testimony of Dr. Risch. He summarized a number of nonrandomized but controlled studies finding HCQ effective for high-risk outpatients.

- 636 outpatients in Sao Paulo, Brazil
- 199 clinic patients in Marseille, France
- 717 patients across a large HMO network in Brazil
- 226 nursing home patients in Marseille
- 1,247 outpatients in New Jersey
- 100 long-term care institution patients in Andorra (between France and Spain)
- 7,892 patients across Saudi Arabia

What's important about these varied study results is that they reflect treatment of high-risk people and that together they all showed a statistically significant benefit of about 50 percent or greater reduction in hospitalization or death.

One study was especially significant. The Saudi Arabia study covered the entire nation and found a five-fold reduction in mortality for HCQ plus zinc versus zinc alone. Moreover, as to safety, not a single fatal cardiac arrhythmia was found among the thousands of patients who could be linked to HCQ.

For the Sao Paulo study, there are some facts worth attention. The outcome used for analysis was a need for hospitalization, defined as a clinically worsening condition or significant shortness of breath (blood oxygen saturation <90%). Even though the severities of all of the recorded influenza-like signs and symptoms and of important comorbid conditions (diabetes, hypertension, asthma, stroke) were substantially greater in the treated patients than in the controls, the need for hospitalization was significantly lower: 1.2 percent in patients starting treatment before day seven of symptoms versus 3.2 percent for patients starting treatment after day seven, showing the importance of early treatment. For the control group the figure was 5.4%, showing the effect of no treatment. No cardiac arrhythmias were reported in the treated patients.

Risch has described a study in a long-term-care facility in Long Island, New York. Of about 200 high-risk patients treated with HCQ plus doxycycline, nine (4.5%) died—a result that is better than generally observed for COVID patients in nursing homes. He also reported in May 2020 the following: Substantial fractions of physicians treating COVID-19 patients (mostly outpatients) in Europe and elsewhere report use of HCQ plus azithromycin: 72% in Spain, 49% in Italy, 41% in Brazil, 39% in Mexico, 28% in France, 23% in the United States, 17% in Germany, 16% in Canada, and 13% in the United Kingdom.

Following are some examples of successful use of HCQ in hospitals to provide more evidence of the efficacy of this medicine for situations where people obviously had enough serious symptoms to be hospitalized. If HCQ has worked often in hospitals, people should have confidence in using it for early home/outpatient treatment long before the COVID disease gets serious enough to require going to a hospital.

A Chinese study reported in April 2020 considered 568 critically ill hospital patients with a median age of sixty-eight; they received a basic treatment including antiviral drugs and antibiotics, and forty-eight of them additionally received HCQ treatment (200 milligrams twice a day for 7-10 days). Primary endpoint was death, and inflammatory cytokines levels were compared between HCQ and non-HCQ treatments. Deaths were 18.8 percent in the HCQ group and 45.8 percent in the non-HCQ group, a stunning nearly 2.5 times higher death rate. The time of hospital stay before patient death was fifteen days and eight days for the HCQ and non-HCQ groups, respectively. It was concluded that HCQ treatment is significantly associated with a decreased mortality in critically ill patients with COVID-19 through attenuation of an inflammatory cytokine storm. Therefore, HCQ should be prescribed for treatment of critically ill COVID-19 patients to save lives.

The HCQ cocktail was also noted to have been standard-of-care treatment for some time at four New York University hospitals, where it was found that adding zinc sulfate significantly cut both intubation and mortality risks by almost half. Now, almost all HCQ protocols include zinc. The study looked at the records of 932 COVID-19 patients treated at local hospitals with hydroxychloroquine and azithromycin. More than 400 of them were also given 100 milligrams of zinc daily. Researchers said the patients given zinc were one and a half times more likely to recover, decreasing their need for intensive care.

A study involving over 100 hospitals in Belgium for hospitalized patients with COVID infection also found positive results, just with using HCQ alone at a dose of 2,400 milligrams over five days. Of 8,075 patients with complete discharge data on 24 May 2020 and diagnosed before 1 May 2020, 4,542 received HCQ in monotherapy and 3,533 were in the no-HCQ group. Death was reported in 804/4,542 (17.7%) and 957/3,533 (27.1%) cases, respectively. Compared with the no-HCQ group, mortality in the HCQ group was reduced both in patients diagnosed ≤5 days (n=3,975) and >5 days (n=3,487) after symptom onset, respectively. The important thing to emphasize is that the 35 percent reduction in death was just for HCQ in this early study, not a cocktail that has become standard for early home/outpatient treatment.

A study reported in July 2020 at the Henry Ford Health System in Michigan received considerable attention. In an analysis of 2,541 patients between March 10 and May 2 across the system's six hospitals, the study found 13 percent of those treated with HCQ alone died, compared to 20.1 percent among those receiving HCQ plus azithromycin, versus 26.4 percent not treated. There was much media coverage of a 50 percent reduction in deaths with use of HCQ. Importantly, 82 percent of their patients received hydroxychloroquine within the first twenty-four hours of admission, and 91 percent within the first forty-eight hours of admission. Again, it should be noted that hospitalized patients were probably significantly symptomatic before hospital admission.

What if a nation first allowed use of HCQ and then blocked its use and then changed policy and restarted its use? This is exactly what was unintentionally done in Switzerland. Use was temporarily suspended on May 27, 2020 for three weeks, and then reinstated. The stoppage was a result of a fraudulent published article that was negative about HCQ and then retracted. During this twenty-day window, a dramatic increase in mortality from COVID-19 was observed, from near zero percent to about 16 percent deaths, which then dropped to a very low value after the reinstatement of HCQ use. This showed causality that removing the drug caused increased mortality from the virus.

Finally, it is important to note a website that provides data on the early use of HCQ. As of late November 2020, some 189 studies on c19study.com showed a median 64 percent reduction in negative virus impacts, hospitalizations, or deaths. Notably, early treatment studies show 100 percent effectiveness. This site lists all the studies it has examined which readers can access.

Another analysis on hcqmeta.com for HCQ found that it is an effective early treatment for COVID-19. "Early treatment is most successful, with 100% of studies reporting a positive effect and an estimated reduction of 65% in the effect measured (death, hospitalization, etc.) using a random effects meta-analysis." The probability that an ineffective treatment generated results, as of December 2020, as positive as the 156 studies to date is estimated to be one in thirty-six trillion.

There have been some cases where reanalysis of data was important. In September 2020, an analysis on the World Tribune website by R. Clinton Ohlers titled, "Effectiveness of hydroxychloroquine was hiding in plain sight," deserved attention. He examined a May 2020 published study that was highly publicized for its negative findings on HCQ for not being effective in New York patients. In truth, what Ohlers revealed was that: "Survival rates for hospitalized patients who received the drug approached 85%" and "with azithromycin the survival rate rose as high as 90%." Without either drug, "survival fell to levels as low as 53%." The conclusion was that the very early study showed "a highly effective, inexpensive, and widely available treatment for COVID-19 is already in hand." This, too, was observed: "It now appears that the disregard of hydroxychloroquine that followed the JAMA publication was gravely premature. Although the authors' own conclusions about the drug were negative, their data actually contains potent indicators of the drug's effectiveness, even when administered under far less than ideal circumstances."

2.3 Clinical experience of courageous American doctors

Dr. Vladimir Zelenko is now recognized as the most significant medical pioneer in the US. He became famous in some medical circles for early use in March 2020 of a HCQ cocktail, including zinc, that cut hospitalizations by 84 percent. It was the inclusion of zinc that was of paramount importance and his recognized innovation. He has spoken of the zinc use as so effective because HCQ and quercetin are zinc ionophores, meaning they get zinc into cells where COVID virus replication can be effectively attacked.

He has treated over 3,000 COVID patients in New York, and has advised other physicians to use his protocol who have treated over 10,000 Americans.

Zelenko emphasizes that all of his outpatients who were considered high risk fully recovered if they received a triple cocktail consisting of HCQ, zinc, and an antibiotic, either azithromycin or doxycycline. It was administered within the first four days of symptoms and taken for at least five days. He has recounted that his high-risk patients included the elderly, some were Holocaust survivors over ninety years old, as well as cancer patients and those with diabetes and other comorbidities. He emphasizes that his group of high-risk patients would be expected to have a fatality rate between 5 percent and 20 percent, but all of the patients had a fatality rate of zero percent!

Moreover, Zelenko emphasizes that his patients have gone on to develop antibodies to COVID-19. His conclusion: His cocktail provides a cure and immunity quickly and inexpensively.

Zelenko has explained why early treatment is critical. It is because COVID-19 is at least a two-phase disease, the first being virus replication and the second being respiratory inflammation, including pneumonia in the lungs. The goal is to quickly stop virus replication and viral shedding and contagion. Otherwise, a patient may need hospitalization to treat lung issues.

He started a petition to the White House in October 2020, naming Fauci and other government officials for blocking HCQ use, noting: "Over 160,000 people were hospitalized and died unnecessarily. Let's make life-saving treatment available and end the pandemic. Let's bring these criminals to justice." "Criminal" is the correct way of seeing the government officials who have blocked early home/outpatient COVID treatment.

Another frontline hero doctor is Brian Tyson in California, who uses an HCQ cocktail, including zinc and an antibiotic, to treat outpatients. He said in October 2020 that he (along with colleague Dr. George Fareed) has cured over 2,000 patients, from eleven months to over ninety years old. "We treated this virus early. We treated this virus aggressively. We only had one hospitalization and zero deaths. Zero deaths, because we were not going to stand by and allow people to die without treatment. We were at the heart of the pandemic due to our large Hispanic and diabetic population. We were told to stop testing. We were told to stop prescribing. But we didn't. We continued to treat patients... We sent them home with treatment. We re-evaluated and every one of them survived," said Tyson.

As a frontline doctor, Tyson said this in October 2020: "This virus has killed people! It will kill more. The question is, how many more will die unnecessarily due to not getting the available treatment? How many will die in fear, and how many will die alone? When you get sick, you do not go to the CDC or the NIH or call the FDA to get diagnosed and treated. You go to your doctor! You go to the people who have seen the disease before and know how to treat it. This virus is no different."

George Fareed, another California doctor, has also found success in treating coronavirus patients with an HCQ cocktail, including azithromycin or doxycycline plus zinc. As reported in July 2020, he said that for three months he had been using the HCQ cocktail to treat patients. He said that the cocktail was "based upon now many studies from colleagues around the world. It's shown to be an effective treatment and that's what we need." He noted that for three months he had been using the HCQ cocktail to treat outpatients. "We need to alleviate the fear in the population that they should know that they can take something that will help them avoid pneumonia and deterioration that we want to see stopped. We've seen thousands of patients and our results have been very favorable," said Fareed.

Dr. Anthony Cardillo in California said he has seen very promising results when prescribing HCQ and zinc for the most severely ill COVID-19 patients. "Every patient I've prescribed it to has been very, very ill and within eight to twelve hours, they were basically symptom-free," Cardillo said. "So clinically I am seeing a resolution," he added.

Dr. Mohammud Alam, in New York, used HCQ and doxycycline. As an infectious disease specialist, he found 81 percent of infected COVID patients he treated at three Long Island nursing homes recovered from the contagion. "In this crisis, I realized I had to do something," Alam said. "I realized if this was my dad, what would I do? And I would do anything I could to help."

Dr. Stephen Smith, founder of The Smith Center for Infectious Diseases and Urban Health in New Jersey, became an early enthusiast on the use of HCQ and azithromycin to treat COVID-19 patients, calling it "a game-changer." At one early point he said he was treating seventy-two COVID-19 patients and that not a single one who had been on that protocol for five days or more had to be intubated. In April 2020, he said, "I think this is the beginning of the end of the pandemic. I'm very serious." This view received national media attention. But then the attack on HCQ made that optimistic forecast a dream, and Smith was also personally attacked. Smith said that he thought his positive results supported the work done in France by Dr. Raoult. He also said that banning a drug [HCQ] when drugs are routinely given off label is "insane."

Dr. Ananda Prasad, a ninety-two-year-old professor, researcher, and hematologist at Wayne State University, and his wife tested positive with COVID-19. Using a combination of HCQ and zinc, both senior patients became free of the virus.

2.4 A unique examination of two classes of nations

Here is a discussion of one of the best sources of information on HCQ as of November 14, 2020. The website hcqtrial.com is titled "Early treatment with hydroxychloroquine: a country-based analysis," in which a very innovative analysis is performed. In those countries with wide early use of HCQ, the death rate is 70 percent lower than in those nations, like the US, where its use has been limited by government. More than 700,000 people have been saved worldwide.

The nine nations in the treatment group that used HCQ are: Costa Rica, Morocco, Ukraine, Russia, Turkey, India, Greece, Algeria, and Cuba, with a total population of 1.8 billion. The average death rate is 368 per million.

On the other side is the control group of nations without wide use of HCQ: Mexico, France, United Kingdom, USA, Netherlands, Sweden, Ireland, and Canada, with a total population of 663 million. The average death rate is 1,221 per million. The average for the whole world is 194.

The site explains that it examined diabetes, obesity, hypertension, life expectancy, population density, urbanization, vaccine use, testing level, and intervention level, which do not account for the effect observed.

You might ask why so relatively few countries are in the two control and treatment groups? Adding credibility to these data are the countries excluded and why they were.

Some were excluded because their population is less than one million. Others because less than 0.5 percent of the population is greater than age eighty. Others were excluded because they quickly adopted widespread mask use. Some were excluded because they have no or very little spread to date.

One thing is clear to anyone objectively examining the data and analysis on this website. It clearly is first rate and worthy of trust and use.

2.5 Prophylactic use of generic medicines and supplements

Though most of the attention has been given to HCQ and various cocktails including it for early home/outpatient COVID treatment, the prophylactic or preventive use of various medicines and supplements has also received attention. In other words, people can choose not to wait until they get COVID symptoms or a positive test. This is the easiest form of home/outpatient treatment, though if you choose to use a prescription medicine, you still need to see a physician willing to prescribe what you want to use.

All of us can take personal initiative to protect our lives, and this can be seen as competitive to taking a vaccine. Considering significant uncertainties about how long immunity lasts with the new COVID vaccines, as well as about effectiveness for older people and those with serious underlying medical conditions, staying with preventive action may be justified.

To begin, this author, based on many months of researching the medical literature, has been using what many others have concluded is a sensible preventive cocktail. For your consideration is the use of these supplements: quercetin, zinc, and vitamin D. The quercetin acts as a substitute for HCQ in that it gets zinc into cells. Typical use is to take a zinc supplement that supplies fifty milligrams; this could be a supplement product such as zinc sulfate labeled as 220 milligrams or a zinc gluconate labeled as fifty milligrams. Quercetin is typically sold as 500 milligrams. Vitamin D is available with 2,000 IU. One or two daily cocktails of one each of the three supplements is a safe and sensible prophylactic cocktail. All of these three supplements have been safely used for many decades.

Dr. Ramin Oskoui has talked about zinc and vitamin D, and says he suggests all his patients take them as prophylaxis. It's "a simple health measure that could be implemented easily." He has expressed dismay as to why supplementation has not been officially recommended.

Indeed, as to the big pandemic blunder, it is somewhat amazing that public health agencies do not work hard at promoting the use of common supplements as a preventive or prophylactic measure against the coronavirus, especially for vulnerable older people and others with serious comorbidities.

Vitamin D in particular has received much attention at the website COVID.us.org, which provides many references for finding evidence that this vitamin reduces the risk of COVID infection. There are some doctors who recommend much higher doses than 2,000 IU once or twice a day, such as 10,000 IU daily. Also, many doctors have advocated taking high doses if one gets COVID symptoms.

A Harvard Medical School publication said this: "Vitamin D may protect against COVID-19 in two ways. First, it may help boost our bodies' natural defense against viruses and bacteria. Second, it may help prevent an exaggerated inflammatory response, which has been shown to contribute to severe illness in some people with COVID-19."

HCQ has also often been advised for use as a preventive medicine, but the problem for Americans is that getting this requires effort, including finding a doctor willing to prescribe it and getting it from foreign sources that do not require a prescription. However, in countries where HCQ is readily available, often as an over-the-counter medicine, prophylactic use has often been widespread. This has been the reported case for India.

Dr. Watanabe from Brazil reanalyzed a June 2020 Minnesota study of adults who had household or occupational exposure to someone with confirmed COVID-19. The study had a negative conclusion. But the new analysis found that for very early preventive HCQ use, there was a "reduction in symptomatic outcomes 72% after 0 days (first day of infection), 48.9% after 1 day and 29.3% after 2 days"—all compared to a placebo group. Conclusion: "Infected patients may have a large benefit if treated as early as possible."

A July 2020 Lancet study, "Hydroxychloroquine Pre-Exposure Prophylaxis for COVID-19 Among Healthcare Workers: Initial Experience from India," found that HCQ use as a prophylaxis for healthcare workers reduced risk of COVID-19 infection by 87 percent. The location was New Delhi, India, and included 334 healthcare workers at risk for contracting COVID-19. The primary study outcome was incidence of adverse effects and efficacy in preventing COVID-19. The HCQ dosage was: 800 milligrams on day one, followed by 400 milligrams once a week. No heart abnormalities were found. Using a weekly dose of 200 to 400 milligrams has been reported in a lot of the literature. The India study conclusion was: "HCQ is safe at the recommended dose for pre-exposure prophylaxis of COVID-19. HCQ chemo-prophylaxis may decrease COVID-19 incidence."

It should also be noted that the India study used only HCQ to reduce risk of infection with COVID-19 without also using zinc. But there have been other studies that have shown zinc increases effectiveness.

Another study, reported in July 2020, described an effort at Baylor University Medical Center, where frontline healthcare workers were given HCQ as a preventive measure. It was completely successful after seven weeks of treatment followed by forty-nine days of follow-up attention after the last dose. The dosing that was considered safe for frontline workers in hospitals and nursing homes was 400 milligrams of HCQ twice on the first day, followed by 200 milligrams twice a day as long as exposure continued.

Another important medicine is ivermectin (IVM), which has also been used as a prophylaxis. IVM is a medication used to treat many types of parasite infestations and came into medical use in 1981. It has been used about 3.8 billion times worldwide, and its success resulted in a 2015 Nobel Prize in medicine. It is also considered an antibiotic and antiviral drug. Like HCL it is a cheap generic requiring a prescription. It is believed that it prevents the coronavirus from entering host cells to stop replication. Dr. Pierre Kory, a frontline doctor dealing with ill COVID patients, has called IVM a "miracle drug" against the COVID disease.

In recent years IVM has been found effective for a number of RNA viruses, including Zika, yellow fever, West Nile, and avian influenza A. COVID-19 is also an RNA virus. So, the repurposing of IVM for the current pandemic makes much sense. But it has not precipitated media attention, thus allowing some doctors at the forefront of the early home/outpatient movement to use IVM effectively. In a sense, use of IVM sidesteps the controversy over HCQ.

A November 2020 review entitled "Review of the Emerging Evidence Demonstrating the Efficacy of Ivermectin in the Prophylaxis and Treatment of COVID-19," from the Front Line COVID-19 Critical Care Alliance, concluded, "In summary, based on the existing and cumulative body of evidence, we recommend the use of ivermectin in both prophylaxis and treatment for COVID-19. In the presence of a global COVID-19 surge, the widespread use of this safe, inexpensive, and effective intervention could lead to a drastic reduction in transmission rates as well as the morbidity and mortality in mild, moderate, and even severe disease phases."

A December 2020 press conference from that group called on "National Health Authorities to Immediately Review Medical Evidence Showing the Efficacy of Ivermectin for the Prevention of COVID-19 and as an Early Outpatient Treatment." Noted at that time was this: "Right now, COVID-19 is a runaway train barreling down the tracks, and if you're on those tracks, ivermectin can help lift you out of harm's way."

Doctors in India have concluded that IVM can be a prophylaxis and a treatment for people infected with the coronavirus, owing to its antiviral properties coupled with effective cost, availability, and good tolerability and safety. In August 2020, the state of Uttar Pradesh in

India announced it was replacing HCQ with IVM (along with doxy-cycline) for preventive treatment of frontline health workers dealing with COVID patients. The protocol was to give the drugs on the first, seventh, and thirtieth day and then once a month.

An interesting case is what happened in a nursing home. The patients were treated with IVM because of an ordinary illness. On one floor residents received a full single dose of probably eighteen milligrams. Other patients were given a lower dose, probably six milligrams. The staff were not treated. Then there was a COVID-19 outbreak. None of the patients on the floor where residents received the higher doses of IVM contracted COVID, even though most of their staff were sick with it. Those who got the lower dose had fewer patients become ill than staff, even though the staff had a much younger median age than the patients, and all the patients had comorbidities.

In Argentina, work in using IVM as a preventive for healthcare workers found that in 800 who received IVM, none got sick with COVID, while for the 400 in the control group, 58 percent got COVID. Dr. Pierre Kory, who recounted this study, said, "We have a solution for this crisis based on mountains of data" and that IVM was a "wonder drug that must be implemented now. IVM should be the standard of care."

On the website hcqmeta.com, the analysis for pre-exposure preventive action found that 79 percent of studies show positive effects, with an estimated reduction of 45 percent in COVID effects.

2.6 New types of American and foreign protocols

IVM has become increasingly used by American doctors for early home/outpatient COVID treatment. The acclaimed Dr. Peter McCullough, noted earlier, has described use of IVM both as an addition to the Zelenko cocktail and as a separate one. For the latter he has described a cocktail of six to twelve milligrams of IVM daily for one to three days, plus an antibiotic such as doxycycline, 100 milligrams twice daily. Depending on symptoms, the cocktail might be used for five or more days.

Dr. Zelenko has also said that because of all the negative "media driven hysteria" about HCQ, he has used IVM in its place in his widely used cocktail.

The website c19study.com presents considerable data on IVM use. It reports that thirty-three studies for early use found 88 percent median improvement, presumably cutting hospitalizations and deaths. All of the studies reported positive results and can be accessed.

As with HCQ, the effectiveness of IVM has been verified in studies of both outpatients and hospital patients. Here are some examples.

A study reported in 2020 titled "Effectiveness of Ivermectin as Add-on Therapy in COVID-19 Management (Pilot Trial)" reported the following: "All the patients of IVM group were cured; none of them died. The mean time to stay in the hospital was significantly lower in IVM group compared with the controls." The hospital time was 7.62 days for IVM versus 13.2 days for control. Results were highly statistically significant.

Another 2020 study involving hospitalized patients in Florida was titled "Ivermectin for COVID-19 Treatment: Clinical Response at Quasi-Threshold Doses Via Hypothesized Alleviation of CD147-Mediated Vascular Occlusion." Results were: "Overall mortality was 15% in the IVM group, 40% less than the 25.2% mortality in the control group. For 75 patients with severe pulmonary disease, those treated with IVM had a mortality of 38.8%, 52% less than the 80.7% mortality in corresponding controls. Stabilization and then improvement often proceeded in 1-2 days, even for patients who had been deteriorating rapidly from room air to supplemental oxygen at up to a 50% mixture."

In July 2020, it was reported that a hospital in Chiapas, Mexico, had success with IVM. It concluded that for outpatients, IVM at twelve milligrams for several days and given at an early state of COVID was 92 percent successful in clearing the virus.

In a December 2020 senate hearing, Dr. Jean-Jacques Rajter said that he had treated hundreds of outpatients with IVM: only two required hospitalization, and none died.

Another study was titled "ICON (Ivermectin in Covid Nineteen) study: Use of Ivermectin Is Associated with Lower Mortality in Hospitalized Patients with COVID-19." It concluded: "Ivermectin was associated with lower mortality during treatment of COVID-19, especially in patients who required higher inspired oxygen or ventilatory support."

Yet another study titled "A comparative observational study on Ivermectin-Doxycycline   and   Hydroxychloroquine-Azithromycin therapy on COVID19 patients" concluded, "Concerning the treatment outcome, adverse effect, and safety, Ivermectin-Doxycycline combination is superior to Hydroxychloroquine-Azithromycin therapy in the case of mild to moderate degree of COVID19 patients."

Doctors in other nations have been active in developing protocols for early home/outpatient use. One example is the work of Dr. Allan Landrito in the Philippines. He recommends a dose of fifteen milligrams of IVM weekly as a preventive measure. For those who are asymptomatic but concerned, he recommends one dose per week for three weeks, and if tested positive up to four weeks. For symptomatic people waiting for a test result he recommends one dose every three to seven days for a maximum of four weeks. For those who are tested positive and have symptoms, the recommendation is the same. In his 2020 *eBook Freedom from COVID-19 Now! – Prevention and Cure at Hand*, Landrito says he has used IVM on over 5,000 patients and that he has "never seen a failure in prevention," suggesting the avoidance of hospitalization.

In September 2020, a news story reported on a treatment developed in Honduras. The Catracho treatment's main components are colchicine (used in some cases to treat swelling, redness, warmth, and pain), tocilizumab (an anti-inflammatory), IVM, blood thinners, and HCQ. The COVID death rate had been reduced by 81.6 percent in thousands of COVID victims.

An article in the *International Journal of Infectious Diseases* in December 2020 described a randomized, double-blind, placebo-controlled trial of oral ivermectin alone (twelve milligrams once daily for five days) or in combination with doxycycline (twelve milligrams ivermectin single dose and 200 milligrams doxycycline day one, followed by 100 milligrams for next four days) compared with placebo among seventy-two hospitalized patients in Dhaka, Bangladesh.

It was noted that "ivermectin, a popular anti-parasitic drug, acts on SARS-CoV-2 by preventing viral proteins from entering the host cell nucleus." The main finding was "in the absence of co-morbidity, a 5-day course of ivermectin treatment showed faster SARS-CoV-2 virus clearance compared to the placebo arm (9 vs.13 days). ...the results provide evidence of the potential benefit of the early intervention with the drug ivermectin for the treatment of adult patients diagnosed with mild SARS-CoV-2. First, early intervention promoted faster viral clearance during disease onset which might have prevented significant immune-system involvement and speed recovery. Secondly, early intervention reduced the viral load faster, thus may help block disease transmission in the general population."

A most interesting study is the prophylactic use of IVM in Peru, titled "Real-World Evidence: The Case of Peru. Causality Between Ivermectin and COVID-19 Infection Fatality Rate," published in October 2020. This study evaluated the impact of IVM interventions from May through September on the excess deaths in people over sixty years old; they generally ranged from about 80 percent to 90 percent death reduction in eight states over two-month periods. Other possible explanations were considered, but the conclusion was that treatment with IVM is the most reasonable explanation for the decrease in number of deaths in Peru. Also, that use of IVM should be public policy, because IVM is a highly effective measure to reduce the excess deaths from COVID-19.

On the website c19ivermectin.com, the analysis found that thirty-four studies of IVM showed 86 percent median improvements for early treatment.

2.7 The myth of randomized clinical trials

What is a randomized clinical trial, or RCT? There is a random allocation of subjects. One group—the experimental group—receives the medicine or intervention being assessed, while the other—the control group—receives an alternative treatment, usually a placebo or no intervention. The groups are monitored to determine the effectiveness and safety of the experimental medicine or intervention relative to the control group. The trial may be blinded, meaning that information which participants have or have not received about the experimental medicine or intervention is withheld until after the trial is complete. This also means that no researchers, technicians, data analysts, or evaluators know who has received the medicine or intervention. Blinding aims to eliminate various kinds of biases.

Observational studies, in which as many patients as possible are treated, have been used in nearly all of the work on examining the effectiveness of HCQ. This is not a matter of choosing a design that is "fatally flawed," as some doctors may charge; rather it is a matter of choosing a design that is not unnecessarily fatal to the patients not chosen for a study. It's not sloppiness (as some critics allege) but being true to the goal of finding a remedy for a disease as quickly as possible. In other words, for pandemic management the fundamental issue is: How soon can we save as many lives as possible? Observational studies can begin almost immediately, and don't require the slow approval process that RCTs require because of government agency regulations and requirements.

When it comes to understanding the limits to RCTs, this article, "Evidence for Health Decision Making—Beyond Randomized, Controlled Trials," August 2017, by Dr. Thomas Frieden, former director of CDC, in the *New England Journal of Medicine*, is widely accepted as a major advance in thinking. Here are some excerpts.

"Elevating RCTs at the expense of other potentially highly valuable sources of data is counterproductive. A better approach is to clarify the health outcome being sought and determine whether existing data are available that can be rigorously and objectively evaluated, independently of or in comparison with data from RCTs, or whether new studies (RCT or otherwise) are needed. ...There is no single, best approach to the study of health interventions; clinical and public health decisions are almost always made with imperfect data. ...There will always be an argument for more research and for better data, but waiting for more data is often an implicit decision not to act or to act on the basis of past practice rather than best available evidence. The goal must be actionable data—data that are sufficient for clinical and public health action that have been derived openly and objectively and that enable us to say, 'Here's what we recommend and why.'"

A key to understanding why the big pandemic blunder has occurred is that the wisdom of Frieden has been ignored, especially by Fauci, who has stubbornly insisted that only RCTs can justify FDA approval for HCQ.

Doidge made this important observation about the COVID pandemic: "Hospitals were finding that 80% of people put on mechanical ventilators died. All the commentators who railed that HCQ was 'unproven' because there had been no randomized control trials (RCTs) didn't mention that standard ventilation treatment for COVID-19, which had become treatment-as-usual overnight for severe cases, had no RCTs supporting it either. There was a double standard as far as HCQ was concerned."

Doidge also noted, "That is one reason why so many researchers, like Raoult, opted for observational studies, in which as many patients as possible are treated. This is not a matter of choosing a design that is 'fatally flawed,' it is a matter of choosing a design that is not unnecessarily fatal to the patients. It's not sloppiness (as some of his critics would allege), but being true to the study question as he saw it: How can we save as many lives as possible. These observational studies could begin almost immediately, and didn't require the slow approval process that RCTs require, in part because of the moral dilemmas they raise. ... Still, given that pandemics kill tens of thousands, if not millions, why not favor the cold-hearted methodologist, who is willing to stand back on a high hill, like a general in a war, and take some casualties to get a win sooner? Isn't that more moral in the long run?"

A NIH website said this about RCTs: "In medicine, it is a problem that is found even in the most respected and cited journals. For instance, a study in *The Journal of the American Medical Association* in 2014, by the Ioannidis group, showed that 35 percent of the conclusions of the finest RCTs, assessed by peer review and published in the most respected medical journals, could not be replicated on reanalysis of their raw data. Meaning that when researchers gave over their original data sets to another group, they could not come up with the same results 35 percent of the time—in the very best, most-cited journals."

A literature review on the representativeness of randomized

controlled trial samples and implications for the external validity of trial results, available on the NIH website, revealed shortcomings of RCTs. It said that one of the weaknesses of RCTs is that in the quest to eliminate confounding factors, they end up, in a majority of cases, excluding patients who are typical of those in the population. The RCT evangelist focuses only on the RCT strengths and forgets their weaknesses. A typical RCT can be helpful in determining what treatment might work for most people in a large population, but not necessarily for specific groups.

Lastly, it is important to recognize that many widely used drugs never had to show positive RCT results, including insulin, tetracycline, prednisone, hydrocortisone, tetanus vaccine, and furosemide (Lasix). This reality seems to be ignored by Fauci, who has stubbornly insisted that a RCT is needed for sanctioning HCQ use.

2.8 More attention needed for federally defined Real World Evidence

Virtually no attention has been given publicly to what was included in the 2016 21st Century Cures Act, particularly section 3022, titled Real World Evidence. Real World Evidence is defined as "data regarding the usage, or the potential benefits or risks, of a drug derived from sources other than randomized clinical trials…including ongoing safety surveillance, observational studies, registries, claims, and patient-centered outcomes research activities…"

The so-called Cures Act also says that Real World Experience may support the approval of new indications for generic drugs. This clearly has extremely important significance for using generic drugs, such as HCQ and IVM, to safely and effectively treat the COVID infection through early home/outpatient treatment.

In other words, this statute provides the legal justification for the FDA not to require RCTs to approve a drug for a particular use. Note that this author's considerable research into what Fauci has said and done has not uncovered any evidence that he understands or in any way uses what the law says about using Real World Evidence.

Importantly, the FDA is authorized to use all of the many types of evidence covered earlier, including many types of retrospective or prospective observational studies, clinical reports and studies, reports by frontline doctors, and analyses of published data. This should have resulted in the FDA's approval of HCQ because of so much evidence for its safety and effectiveness against the coronavirus.

There was important information in a December 2016 article in the *New England Journal of Medicine* titled "Real World Evidence – What Is It and What Can It Tell Us?" All twelve authors were from the FDA. This was said: "We believe that when the term 'real-world evidence' is used, the primary attribute that distinguishes it from other kinds of evidence is related to the context in which the evidence is gathered—in other words, in clinical care and home or community settings as opposed to research-intensive or academic environments. … In order to assess patient outcomes and to ensure that patients get treatment that is right for them, real-world data needs to be utilized."

Here is what must be recognized by public health officials: "Real World Evidence comes into play when clinical trials cannot really account for the entire patient population of a particular disease. Patients suffering from comorbidities or belonging to a distant geographic region or age limit who did not participate in any clinical trial may not respond to the treatment in question as expected. RWE provides answers to these problems and also to analyze effects of drugs over a longer period of time."

A pandemic that is being blamed for huge numbers of hospitalizations and deaths clearly justifies use of Real World Evidence for the use of many documented protocols for early home/outpatient treatment as well as prophylactic use by people.

The long-lasting attack by the media and others against HCQ goes against this view and should be condemned because it is against the letter and spirit of what was put into the federal law. A lot of talk about following the science is empty and dangerous rhetoric. Following the science legally means going way beyond RCTs and should include Real World Evidence. Should attacks begin against IVM, the same would be true to defend its use against COVID.

So, what has FDA said officially relative to all this? "In recent years, the agency has taken steps to leverage modern, rigorous analyses of real-world data—such as data from the health care setting—to inform our work. The COVID-19 pandemic has brought an urgency to these efforts and the FDA has worked quickly to advance collaborations with public and private partners to collect and analyze a variety of real-world data sources. Evaluation of real-world data has the potential to provide a wealth of rapid, actionable information to better understand disease symptoms, describe and measure immunity and understand available medical product supplies to help mitigate potential shortages. These data can also inform ongoing work to evaluate potential therapies, vaccines or diagnostics for COVID-19." This was in "Advancing the

Science of Real-World Data to Address the COVID-19 Pandemic" issued in September 2020. Talk is cheap. Action has not happened.

Clearly, the movement for early home/outpatient COVID treatment should explicitly attack the FDA for not doing what is appropriate and necessary in the pandemic, according to law. But, so far, its failure to do what is right and necessary justifies talking about the big pandemic blunder.

On the international scene, the document "Strengthening global collaboration on COVID-19 real-world evidence and observational studies" by the European Medicines Agency, October 2020, said, "Real-world evidence generated by observational studies is fundamental to understanding the benefits and risks of medicines when used in clinical practice for the prevention and treatment of COVID-19."

Government has not been the only American establishment power to avoid using properly the Real World Evidence mandate in law. There was an April 2020 "Joint statement on ordering, prescribing or dispensing COVID-19 medications – Joint statement of the American Medical Association, American Pharmacists Association and American Society of Health-System Pharmacists." This sent a threat to doctors trying innovative protocols, mostly at this early time using HCQ. It said, "We caution hospitals, health systems, other entities, and individual practitioners that no medication has been FDA-approved for use in COVID-19 patients. Definitive evidence for the role of these drugs in treating COVID-19 patients has not been determined through robust clinical trials; decisions to use these medications off-label must be made with extreme caution and careful monitoring."

After referring to HCQ, this was also stated: "We applaud the ongoing efforts to conduct clinical trials and generate evidence related to these and other medications during a time of pandemic." Absent was recognition of positive evidence as observational patient data coming from clinical use (not formal trials) of HCQ protocols by frontline doctors, such as Dr. Zelenko and Dr. Tyson, that followed pioneering work in France.

Part 3

——∿∿——

Understanding What Has Caused and Shaped the Pandemic Blunder

3.1 Powerful forces block early home/ outpatient COVID treatment

Nearly every part of the political, government, medical, public health, traditional media, and social media establishments and systems have been extremely focused, or more correctly *obsessed*, with the negative aspects of the pandemic.

When there is positive attention or coverage, it is almost always linked to compliance with contagion controls (but not nearly comparable to negative news because of noncompliance)—pillar two, new therapeutics and treatments for hospitalized patients—pillar three, and anticipated power of vaccines to curb the magnitude of the pandemic—pillar four.

Nearly all of the information and news reaching the public represent suppression of good news about pillar one, early home/outpatient treatment. To some degree there has also been a lot of coverage of studies that give negative results about the medicines and protocols used for early home/outpatient treatment. This amounts to disinformation aimed at damping down or completely blocking interest in early home/outpatient treatments that, as presented in Part 2 of this book, considerable data say really are effective.

Is it also useful, as in a worst possible scenario about the COVID pandemic, to contemplate that there has been an intentional scam or hoax perpetrated on the public? If so, has this been done to use the pandemic to give power to a multitude of government local, state, and federal officials to control the lives of Americans? Possibly. The use of authoritarian and unconstitutional contagion controls seen by many people definitely support this view. All kinds of mandates coming from local and state officials have come to be seen correctly by millions of Americans as arbitrary and capricious, and certainly not based on good scientific data. Especially with respect to school closings and lockdowns killing incredible numbers of restaurants, for example.

In November 2020, one person with terrific medical credentials offered a very negative view of what the pandemic really is. He is Dr. Roger Hodkinson, a Canadian. He received his general medical degrees from Cambridge University in the UK. Following a residency at the University of British Columbia, he became a Royal College certified general pathologist (FRCPC) and also a Fellow of the College of American Pathologists (FCAP). He is in good standing with the College of Physicians and Surgeons of Alberta, and has been recognized by the Court of Queen's Bench in Alberta as an expert in pathology. He is also the CEO of a biotech company that manufactures COVID tests.

Noting his credentials is so important because of what he has said publicly. A full transcript of his interview is on the website lifesitenews. com. "There is utterly unfounded public hysteria driven by the media and politicians; it's outrageous; this is the greatest hoax ever perpetrated on an unsuspecting public," said Hodkinson.

Moreover, the doctor said that nothing could be done to stop the spread of the virus besides protecting older, more vulnerable people and that the whole situation represented "politics playing medicine, and that's a very dangerous game."

On specific contagion controls, Hodkinson said, "Social distancing is useless because COVID is spread by aerosols which travel thirty meters or so before landing." This is a lot more than the six feet government agencies refer to. Hodkinson also slammed mandatory mask mandates as completely pointless. "Masks are utterly useless. There is no evidence base for their effectiveness whatsoever," he said. "Paper masks and fabric masks are simply virtue signaling. They're not even worn effectively most of the time. It's utterly ridiculous. Seeing these unfortunate, uneducated people—I'm not saying that in a pejorative sense—seeing these people walking around like lemmings obeying without any knowledge base to put the mask on their face."

The doctor has also criticized the unreliability of PCR tests, noting that "positive test results do not, underlined in neon, mean a clinical infection," and that…the false numbers are "driving public hysteria."

Consistent with what was said in the previous Part 2 discussion, he also called for protecting the vulnerable such as those in nursing homes by giving them "3,000 to 5,000 international units of vitamin D every day, which has been shown to radically reduce the likelihood of infection."

This is how Hodkinson summed things up about all the pandemic actions: "I'm absolutely outraged that this has reached this level; it should all stop tomorrow."

You may think that these are extreme viewpoints, but there are a great many medical professionals who share these views, although most are too concerned about negative impacts of going public with such views. Despite there being strong scientific merit to the views expressed by Hodkinson, he has received considerable criticisms from many establishment groups. His response: "I adamantly stand by my statements."

The bottom line for Hodkinson is also compatible with the thinking of many others, namely the call for society to be re-opened immediately to stop and remedy the debilitating damage being caused by lockdowns. As presented earlier, this is consistent with the Great Barrington Declaration.

3.2 Federal agencies block doctors, restrict care, and feed a conspiracy

The refusal by NIH to provide guidance for using pillar one treatment and the continued blocking of HCQ use by the FDA define a massive national strategy to hold back support for using what has been detailed in the previous part of this book.

The eminent Dr. Peter McCullough got it right in an op-ed article in *The Hill* in August 2020, titled, "Why doctors and researchers need access to hydroxychloroquine." "On July 6, a team of doctors from Henry Ford Hospital, supported by physicians from Baylor University Medical Center, submitted an urgent request to the Food and Drug Administration (FDA) to reauthorize use of hydroxychloroquine (HCQ) for early treatment of COVID-19. Since that day, more than 25,000 more Americans have died from the virus as COVID-19 continues to burn through communities across America. If the results of a recent Henry Ford Hospital study are accurate, at least half of these patients might have been saved by HCQ. ... HCQ was singled out as a political football early in spring—right after President Trump urged the medical community to consider HCQ." FDA refused to save lives.

McCollough also noted this: "The politicization of HCQ is an ongoing tragedy. The Federal Emergency Management Agency (FEMA) has more than 60 million HCQ tablets sitting in its warehouses. Absent a new Emergency Use Authorization, FEMA cannot ship this valuable medicine for appropriate 'off-label' treatment of COVID-19 patients." The HCQ stockpile remains unused as of December 2020. A lawsuit against FDA to free up the stockpile by the American Association of Physicians and Surgeons failed. The group noted FDA officials "care more about their power over the HCQ stockpile than the lives being lost daily without access to it."

Several formal requests to the FDA for emergency use authorization (EUA) for HCQ failed. Here is some important information on EUAs.

The FDA can grant an EUA to a drug to treat COVID-19 and

facilitate the distribution of new therapeutics when there are no alternatives. Many have speculated that the refusal to approve HCQ was motivated by FDA interest in removing an "alternative" that would make granting EUAs to other drugs more difficult. EUAs are important tools during the early stages of any pandemic because they loosen restrictions on novel treatment options. But one issue is that they interfere with clinical trials that would provide the best evidence on whether these drugs are safe and effective.

The EUA means it is "reasonable to believe" that the drug "may be effective." This "may be effective" standard is a much lower level of evidence compared to the "effectiveness" standard the FDA uses for drug approvals.

Not receiving much attention is the fact that there are over thirty American medical societies or organizations that almost entirely follow what the three top federal agencies dealing with the pandemic say and do: NIH, FDA, and CDC, all in the Department of Health and Human Services. They have chosen deliberately to not provide support for early home/outpatient COVID treatment including preventive actions by people, as discussed previously. This is why most American physicians, no matter what their work settings, do not provide their patients any of the large array of medicines and protocols detailed previously. Note that an attempt to change the policy of the largest society, the American Medical Association, and reverse its position against HCQ failed in November 2020.

The net result is that the traditional medical freedom of doctors to treat their patients as they best determine has been wiped out by all levels of government actions, including the whole public health system.

A "Petition For Medical Freedom" was initiated by the United Medical Freedom Super PAC; a letter was sent to many senior federal officials as well as state governors. Here are some excerpts:

"Various agencies, such as the FDA, FTC, CDC, NIH, state licensing boards and state pharmacy boards have inserted themselves between the physicians of this country and their patients who are seeking treatment for COVID-19 illness. Physicians have been trained for years and know their patients better than any federal or state agencies. Physicians should have the right to treat their patients as they see fit and as they have clinically assessed each individual, without governmental interference or fear of retribution.

"Recently the Federal Trade Commission (FTC) sent cease-and-desist letters to hundreds of licensed doctors across the country. These physicians are being threatened with legal action from the FTC if they discuss with patients, or anyone, what they have researched, discovered, and experienced as beneficial for patients with COVID-19 illness. The FTC is therefore practicing medicine without a license, which disrupts the patient/physician decision-making process.

"Governors, often covertly in conjunction with state pharmacy boards, have made it very difficult or impossible for patients to get filled their COVID-19 prescriptions, which are written by physicians properly licensed by their state medical boards. Such governors and pharmacy boards are inserting themselves into the patient-physician relationship.

"There have been statements made to the media and the public by representatives of the National Institutes of Health and the Food and

Drug Administration that US doctors should not treat COVID-19 outpatients prior to the completion of randomized, controlled trials (RCT) showing the benefit of outpatient treatment of COVID-19.

"Unless we put Medical Freedom into the Constitution, the time will come when medicine will organize into an undercover dictatorship. To restrict the art of healing to one class of men and deny equal privileges to others will constitute the bastille of medical science. All such laws are un-American and despotic...The Constitution of the Republic should make special provisions for Medical Freedom as well as Religious Freedom."

This prescient statement surely has not been seen by many Americans. It was written by Dr. Benjamin Rush, George Washington's personal doctor, a signer of the Declaration of Independence, Surgeon General of the Continental Army, and Fellow of the American Academy of Arts and Sciences.

Here is the critical point. When doctors lose their medical freedom, so do patients. Medical liberty is destroyed for American society. This means ordinary people suffer inadequate COVID care because both the health care and public health systems fail them. The fact that death rates from COVID are generally low on average, less than about 1 percent, does not tell the whole story. For those who must go to hospital, even if they survive, they and their loved ones go through a lot of pain and suffering, and COVID victims may have bad long-term effects of the disease progressing past the initial virus replication phase. That is why early treatment is so important.

Everything the government has done nourishes and sustains what can be viewed as a vast national conspiracy. The word "conspiracy" has taken on a negative connotation. But whether or not there are centrally directed actions and explicit communications, it is fair to see what has transpired as a conspiracy of like-minded people in authority to effectively shape public knowledge about the pandemic, as well as control medical treatments.

This broad, national effort by so many power actors and elites has created the big pandemic blunder. Meaning that pillar one, early home/outpatient treatment is kept mostly invisible, no matter how strongly innovative frontline physicians attempt to get their good news out about their clinical experience. In many cases, actions by these courageous doctors have been blocked on social media and not just ignored by the leftist mainstream media.

As to what the government and its allies have done, it is important to understand that so much of the data they emphasize do not warrant public trust. For example, consider what the distinguished Stanford University professor John Ioannidis (an expert in medicine, epidemiology, population health, biomedical data science, and statistics) has said. He is quite famous for his article "Why Most Published Research Findings Are False."

As to the COVID pandemic he said:

"The data collected so far on how many people are infected and how the epidemic is evolving are utterly unreliable. Given the limited testing to date, some deaths and probably the vast majority of infections due to SARS-CoV-2 are being missed. We don't know if we are failing to capture infections by a factor of three or 300…Patients who have been tested for SARS-CoV-2 are disproportionately those with severe symptoms and bad outcomes. As most health systems have limited testing capacity, selection bias may even worsen in the near future."

"The numbers are almost meaningless," says Steve Goodman, a professor of epidemiology at Stanford University. "There's a huge reservoir of people who have mild cases, and would not likely seek testing," he says. "The rate of increase in positive results reflects a mixed-up combination of increased testing rates and spread of the virus."

If you cannot trust government data, then why trust their refusal to support early home/outpatient COVID treatment?

A September 2020 CDC publication gave informative data on HCQ prescriptions at retail stores (not mail order). The prescriptions showed an eighty-fold increase from March 2019 to March 2020, surely due to use for fighting COVID infections. In March through June 2020, there likely were 680,000 HCQ prescriptions for treating the virus, an average of 170,000 per month. However, after the government clamp-down by the FDA, prescriptions in May and June dropped to an average of 80,000 a month. This change might explain increased death rates as many frontline doctors stopped prescribing HCQ for COVID patients.

Here is a key question. Is there a de facto leader of the movement or conspiracy against pillar one options? A person with enough power to shape the actions and commitments of all parts of the national system addressing the pandemic? A person who has been given the power mainly through endless, daily media attention to engender public trust and confidence? A person who receives daily adoration by the leftist media and high-level government officials? A person who uses both behind-the-scenes government power and public exposure and engagement to perpetuate the crisis mentality of the pandemic? The answer is yes to all these questions.

That person is Dr. Anthony Fauci of the NIH, who wields enormous power to suppress pillar one from receiving strong public, government, and media support. More about him follows.

3.3 Fauci has the power and is the main culprit

As mentioned earlier, Fauci has been the director of the National Institute of Allergy and Infectious Diseases at the US National Institutes of Health for thirty-six years. The first thing to emphasize is that diverse actions have made Fauci far more immune from criticism than the public is immune from the coronavirus.

The US leftist mainstream news media has worked to create an image for Fauci as a unique, nation-saving, neutral scientist, physician, and public health expert. The public has been snookered. He has made himself the king of virus medicine through constant media appearances far beyond what is normal for a medical researcher. What the media seems unable to remember is that he is part of a research organization, not a public health or drug approval agency. As much a tyrant as a virus expert, Fauci has stubbornly refused to admit his big mistakes, namely not supporting HCQ use nor early home/outpatient treatment to catch the coronavirus in its first replication stage.

It is wise to see media-crazy Fauci as a narcissist who is routinely terrorizing the public with talk about expensive medicines for hospital patients and vaccines and peddling fear by talking about 300,000 to 400,000 deaths. It appears that Fauci has Narcissistic Personality Disorder, which is characterized by an increased sense of self-importance and excessive urge for admiration. Such an individual has trouble taking criticism, which certainly appears true for Fauci.

The eminent Dr. Peter McCullough got it right in his op-ed article in August 2020. "HCQ was singled out as a political football early in spring. … [Fauci's] opposition has become a rallying cry of the left-leaning mainstream media's 'Hydroxy Hysteria.' The politicization of HCQ is an ongoing tragedy."

What Fauci has mostly been, in fact, is a remarkably successful bureaucrat for his multibillion-dollar operation. He is also a brilliant manipulator of the media to create and sustain a popular image that hardly anyone is willing to attack during the pandemic. He is a master of staying in the public limelight through television, radio, and newspaper interviews, and a constant presence on many websites. Conference after conference gets Fauci to be a main speaker. It is a full-time job to stay in the public limelight, to ensure that any article or show on the pandemic features Fauci.

What few people understand is that Fauci also has a political agenda. So much of what he does and says in a very public way has supported the massive anti-Trump movement, especially in the mainstream news media, which is remarkably liberal and Democrat Party oriented. Anti-Trump media has successfully cloaked Fauci in a myth of a public health expert, the ultimate and final arbiter of what is needed to fight the pandemic. In fact, what is hidden from the public is that his views and actions have resulted in hundreds of thousands of deaths from the virus. Countless numbers of people who have suffered awful medical distress and economic pain remain ignorant of the very dark side of Fauci if they depend on leftist mainstream news.

In a world where true justice prevailed, Fauci would be prosecuted for crimes against humanity for preventing widespread pillar one medicines and protocols that could have, and still can, prevent countless deaths. This started when Fauci decided to condemn the use of HCQ and get the NIH to prevent any action for home/outpatient COVID treatment.

A most important analysis on the Real Clear Politics website was an original essay (unusual for this website to publish) in August 2020, titled "An Effective COVID Treatment the Media Continues to Besmirch" by Steven Hatfill, a highly respected physician and veteran virologist.

It noted that "the 'Fauci Strategy' was to keep early infected patients quarantined at home without treatment until they developed a shortness of breath and had to be admitted to a hospital. ... The Food and Drug Administration cluelessly agreed to this doctrine and it stated in its hydroxychloroquine Emergency Use Authorization (EUA) that 'hospitalized patients were likely to have a greater prospect of benefit (compared to ambulatory patients with mild illness).' In reality just the opposite was true. This was a tragic mistake by Fauci and FDA Commissioner Dr. Stephen Hahn. It was a mistake that would cost the lives of thousands of Americans in the days to come."

Here is more of what the insightful Hatfill said: "When the COVID-19 pandemic began, a search was made for suitable antiviral therapies to use as treatment until a vaccine could be produced. One drug, hydroxychloroquine, was found to be the most effective and safe for use against the virus. …there was no guidance from Dr. Anthony Fauci or the NIH Treatment Guidelines Panel on what role the drug would play in the national pandemic response. Fauci seemed to be unaware that there actually was a national pandemic plan for respiratory viruses. Following a careful regimen developed by doctors in France, some knowledgeable practicing US physicians began prescribing hydroxychloroquine to patients still in the *early phase* of COVID infection. Its effects seemed dramatic. Patients still became sick, but for the most part they avoided hospitalization. In contrast—and in error—the NIH-funded studies somehow became focused on giving hydroxychloroquine to late-presenting hospitalized patients. This was in spite of the fact that unlike the drug's early use in ambulatory patients, there was no real data to support the drug's use in more severe hospitalized patients." Hatfill got this exactly right and recognized the pioneering efforts of Dr. Zelenko and a few other American doctors.

Hatfill correctly noted more about the history of bad Fauci and government thinking: "Accumulating data showed remarkable results if hydroxychloroquine were given to patients early, during a seven-day window from the time of first symptom onset. If given during this window, most infections did not progress into the severe, lethal second stage of the disease. Patients still got sick, but they avoided hospitalization or the later transfer to an intensive care unit. In mid-April a high-level memo was sent to the FDA alerting them to the fact that the best use for hydroxychloroquine was for its early use in still ambulatory COVID patients. These patients were quarantined at home but were not short of breath and did not yet require supplemental oxygen and hospitalization. Failing to understand that COVID-19 could be a two-stage disease process, the FDA ignored the memo and it withdrew its

EUA for hydroxychloroquine based on flawed studies and clinical trials that were applicable only to late-stage COVID patients."

This was a horrendously poor government decision that to this day explains why there has been no wide use of early home/outpatient COVID treatment that could keep people healthy and out of the hospital.

Even after increasing evidence that HCQ was effective, Hatfill noted, "Fauci continued to ignore the ever accumulating and remarkable early-use data on hydroxychloroquine and he became focused on a new antiviral compound named remdesivir. This was an experimental drug that had to be given intravenously every day for five days. It was never suitable for major widespread outpatient or at-home use as part of a national pandemic plan. We now know that remdesivir has no effect on overall COVID patient mortality and it costs thousands of dollars per patient. Hydroxychloroquine, by contrast, costs 60 cents a tablet, it can be taken at home, it fits in with the national pandemic plan for respiratory viruses." Clearly, Hatfill at an early time correctly assessed the potential for pillar one emphasis, though at the time it was only HCQ getting attention, and not the multi-ingredient cocktail approach, usually including zinc and an antibiotic like doxycycline.

If you accept the abundant evidence that hydroxychloroquine is both an effective preventive as well as a cure when prescribed by doctors at an early point, especially before hospitalization, then you begin to understand why Fauci has blood on his hands. It is reasonable to hope that an accurate historical analysis of this pandemic will show this, just as Hatfill accurately analyzed in August 2020.

In September 2020, Jordan Schachtel summed up things nicely in his article "Mad scientist: Fauci demands total U.S. shutdown until COVID vaccine arrives." "There is no basis for Fauci's claim that he can manipulate society into stopping the virus. He is either a victim of the illusion of control, or he has embraced total deception as part of his power drunk campaign to stay in the spotlight," he said. He also said that Fauci had ignored "the devastating side effects of his favored heavy-handed approaches. The economic and societal ramifications from his implemented COVID lockdowns have devastated millions of American families, putting millions out of work, and millions more into positions of severe hardship, all to combat a virus with a 99.8% recovery rate." Also, Fauci was "continuing with his fearmongering, pseudoscience campaigns." Exactly right.

3.4 Exactly what is wrong with Fauci

Few medical professionals speak publicly about Fauci. Why? With his huge annual budget of nearly $6 billion, he dispenses about $4 billion a year to outside people and groups. Many physicians and epidemiologists have widely divergent professional opinions. But they fear talking about Fauci and losing financial support. Three frontline doctors sent a detailed letter in August 2020 to Fauci with many serious questions. But Fauci did not respond. One of those doctors observed "rigorous questioning of Dr. Fauci with challenges from his peers has never occurred. Dr. Fauci's opinions remain not only unchallenged, but those with opposing views are censored."

But people in the conservative arena have been finding fault with Fauci. Here are some examples of insightful criticism.

Don't be fooled by his grandfather demeanor. Recognize that he is a subversive collaborator with the leftist media campaign against President Trump. Worse, as a physician he has failed his oath to first do no harm. Daily, the mainstream media treats Fauci as a deity, but there have been some critics with wise observations, mostly in conservative media. These views counter the propaganda of the mainstream media.

Jim Hoft on The Gateway Pundit website said: "From the beginning of this pandemic Fauci has been completely misguided and inaccurate in his predictions and treatment of the Chinese COVID-19 virus."

Brent Smith on the WND website asked the right question: "How does Dr. Anthony Fauci still have a job? He's part of the Inside-the-Beltway Deep State and has attempted to undermine the president since he was elevated to the position of Doctor COVID Know-it-All."

Thomas Lifson on The American Thinker website made this wise observation: "The suppression of the use of hydroxychloroquine in combination with zinc to treat COVID-19 amounts to the biggest public health scandal since the Tuskegee Study."

Stacey Lennox on the PJ Media website correctly noted: "Every possible outpatient treatment from HCQ to inhaled corticosteroids has been suppressed or ignored by the NIH and FDA and Dr. Fauci specifically. This dismissal of early outpatient treatment is unconscionable as is the suppression and silencing of clinicians who have observational data to share from caring for actual patients."

On the FDA stopping HCQ use, Dr. Kristin Held, president of the American Association of Physicians and Surgeons, said it "contributed to increased COVID cases and death.... Who bears responsibility for such evil? ...Dr. Fauci failed us. We were not prepared, and preparedness was his charge. He can no longer be trusted."

There is a good case for thinking of Fauci as a new kind of war criminal. This fits with the view that the US has been fighting a war against the China coronavirus. There are valid reasons for believing that Fauci has violated public trust in him because he has willfully deceived the public.

What explains his behavior? Fauci has a long history of being very close to the Chinese Communist Party (CCP) and the World Health Organization (WHO). WHO has been in the pocket of the CCP and played a key role in letting the pandemic loose on the world. It also has not done what it could have in promoting global use of HCQ. Fauci helped steer US funding for creating the Wuhan lab that let loose the CCP virus and has been proud of working with Chinese scientists while ignoring that they are beholden to the CCP.

Also note on January 21, 2020 in the *Washington Post,* Fauci said the CCP virus "is not a major threat for the people of the United States and this is not something that the citizens of the United States right now should be worried about." In fact, toward the end of December 2019 and early in January 2020, there was evidence that a very dangerous, contagious virus had been unleashed from China, though WHO ignored the evidence.

Another aspect of Fauci's failing is that he stubbornly dismissed a great many studies and test results showing the efficacy and safety of HCQ by only supporting extensive, lengthy, randomized, placebo-controlled, double-blind studies. As discussed previously, many doctors have noted there are countless highly used prescription medicines that have never gone through such lengthy and expensive three-phase testing. Why has Fauci stubbornly refused to acknowledge and accept the positive findings from all kinds of other studies by clinicians in the US and a number of other countries?

As noted on Bloomberg News in August 2020, Fauci said that health experts are unanimous about this medicine, meaning his view that HCQ was ineffective. This was a total lie. You have to wonder why he would proclaim such a wrong statement in the face of many published writings indicating just the opposite. The obvious explanation is that he wants to purposefully mislead the public and attack the great many physicians advocating the early use of HCQ.

Here is an important example of Fauci's leftist mindset. It is hard to understand Fauci's July 2020 praising of New York State's handling of the pandemic on a National Public Radio interview. This was long after widespread condemnation of its incredibly high death rate. This also illustrates the sheer ego and belief of being immune to public criticism that defines Fauci. Leftist views and propaganda were addressed by Dennis Prager, who aptly said leftists had "weaponized medicine."

A most important aspect of Fauci's leftist proclivity was revealed in the July 2020 PJ Media website article "Dr. Fauci: 'There's No Inconsistency' in Banning Church and Business But Allowing Mass Protests." This was the big point: "During a House Judiciary Committee hearing on Friday, Rep. Jim Jordan (R-Ohio) pressed Dr. Anthony Fauci on whether the government should restrict the massive Black Lives Matter protests across the country in order to slow the spread of the coronavirus. Fauci admitted that crowds full of people not wearing masks would likely spread the virus, but he refused to say whether or not protests would do so. He also refused to make any recommendations on limiting protests, even though he had made many recommendations in the past."

In a similar vein, in an article in *The Washington Examiner* in October 2020, Emma Colton put Fauci on the spot by getting him to refuse to criticize a large leftist women's march as a virus-spreading event, in contrast to his widely spread comment criticizing a rather small White House event.

In other words, the constantly pontificating Fauci chose not to criticize leftist street activities even though they clearly did not follow his sacred contagion controls.

In a similar vein, in October 2020, as soon as candidate Biden talked about a national mandate for masks, Fauci said on news shows it would be a "great idea" to have a national mask mandate. Surely he knew that the federal government had no such power; it was up to states.

A very important point to make about Fauci is that he poses as a public health official, but does not fully acknowledge all the negative impacts of actions he advocates. Particularly, he ignores many negative health impacts from contagion controls, especially lockdowns that seriously harm American society and economy. Neither is Fauci an epidemiologist. Trained as a physician, he is a super-bureaucrat who has largely supplanted the CDC, the Surgeon General, and the FDA.

On the ProPublica.org website it was revealed in the October 2020 article "Who Decides When Vaccine Studies Are Done? Internal Documents Show Fauci Plays a Key Role" that Fauci has the power to control whether a vaccine gets approved or not, though it appears to the public that the FDA has that power. It noted, "Dr. Anthony Fauci will see data from government-funded vaccine trials before the FDA does." This also was noted: "Fauci's role in overseeing the companies that are participating in Operation Warp Speed arises from a unique arrangement that the government set up to monitor the trials. Typically, clinical trials set up their own independent panels of scientists, known as a data safety monitoring board or DSMB, to watch out for safety concerns or early signs of success. But all of the vaccine trials in Operation Warp Speed are sharing a common DSMB whose members were selected by Fauci's agency, the NIAID."

3.5 The corruption of money

A great example of how money and greed have corrupted pandemic management by the government is the case of the patented, high-priced drug remdesivir, used for hospital patients and given to President Trump, noted by Hatfill.

An inevitable, logical, and necessary question to consider is exactly why has Fauci chosen to sacrifice the lives of so many people by dismissing the benefits of hydroxychloroquine at a very early time in the pandemic, and even now? And why has he championed remdesivir?

Fauci for decades has had close relationships with the largest global pharmaceutical companies. A main reason was his work years ago on fighting the AIDS epidemic, for which a number of new drugs became successful treatment. Blocking widescale use of extremely low-cost generic medicines like HCQ and IVM is key to safeguarding trillions of dollars to be made for worldwide treatment drugs, therapeutics, and vaccines for the COVID pandemic.

A big example is Gilead Sciences Inc., which produces remdesivir. It said it would charge US hospitals $3,120 per patient with typical commercial insurance. It is for critically ill patients in hospitals only. As said by Hatfill, "Hydroxychloroquine, by contrast, costs 60 cents a tablet, it can be taken at home, it fits in with the national pandemic plan for respiratory viruses, and a course of therapy simply requires swallowing three tablets in the first 24 hours followed by one tablet every 12 hours for five days."

Fauci's group ran the key study on remdesivir and publicly proclaimed positive results before the results were peer reviewed and published in a medical journal. So much for scientific integrity. The government spent at least $70.5 million of taxpayer money on its development. He got the drug approved before usual phase 3 testing was completed, and paid for the clinical trial. Significantly, the NIH advisory panel that reviewed remdesivir for the FDA had, among fifty-four scientific panel members, eighteen with financial ties to pharma companies.

During 2020, articles appeared highlighting the competition between HCQ and remdesivir to fight the pandemic. But the competition was lopsided, like a kite competing against a jet plane. Why? So much money and so many powerful people pushing remdesivir. So little money to be made from using HCQ.

What about the medical and scientific proof? It is like night and day. Remdesivir has only been shown to modestly reduce hospital time by a few days. In contrast, as shown previously, HCQ in countless studies has been shown to cut hospitalizations and deaths. When remdesivir was in clinical studies, the government (Fauci) and Gilead cleverly changed what measured outcome effectiveness. The protocol was changed after the trial started, a very unorthodox procedure. Rather than measure death, the length of hospital stay, a far less rigorous measure, was deemed to determine success against COVID-19. Why? Because remdesivir did not reduce the death rate significantly. With billions of dollars at stake, they needed a way to make the drug a market success, despite a cost of thousands of dollars per patient.

Data on remdesivir just published by the University of Minnesota showed it "had little effect in patients with moderate COVID-19 in 105 hospitals in the United States, Europe, and Asia in a randomized, controlled trial...adding to a mixed picture of the drug in randomized clinical trials (RCTs), which are considered the gold standard for gauging interventions." Similarly, a physician on an emergency medicine blog, rebelem.com, presented a detailed analysis and concluded, "Combining all the evidence we have thus far, remdesivir is far from a savior in COVID-19."

In a strange coincidence of timing, the same day that news hit about Trump catching the virus, *The Washington Post* had a major story in September 2020 with the headline "Remdesivir may not cure coronavirus, but it's on track to make billions for Gilead." What first appears as a puff piece promoting remdesivir reveals on close reading a number of points that should shake up people.

Here are some examples:

An official with the Association of American Medical Colleges pointed out the "flattening demand" and "If it prevented people from dying, there would be a different demand."

A noted clinician and researcher said, "Remdesivir is not the answer to the epidemic. It's going to play a role in helping a few people."

Fauci was said to declare remdesivir a "modest weapon against the disease but said it would be the standard of care." But such a standard would not apply to the multitude of people not in a hospital. Without allowing a standard of care for HCQ, it is largely doomed.

Another physician spoke of the drug probably offering "some benefit."

The Post noted that the drug "reduces hospital stays from 15 to 11 days but does not significantly reduce the odds of dying of the coronavirus."

Dr. Mark Siedner, an infectious disease expert at Massachusetts General Hospital, said, "Remdesivir is not the answer to the epidemic. It's going to play a role in helping a few people. Is it going to help us in lockdowns, school closures and cancellation of football seasons? Absolutely not."

As to granting standard of care recognition for remdesivir, it has been noted on the Federalist website in August 2020 that the National Institutes of Health (NIH) panel had members with financial ties to the manufacturer, Gilead, and that the same panel ruled against HCQ as a standard of care.

In May 2020 on The National Interest website, the article "Head to Head: Is Chloroquine or Remdesivir the Drug to Treat Coronavirus?" noted correctly that "there is no fair test of the two top contending treatments being conducted." Fauci was clearly seen as a promoter of remdesivir. And, just as more work would show, this article correctly noted the serious side effect, namely "abnormal liver function."

Indeed, the European drugs regulator said that its safety committee was reviewing reports of acute kidney injury in some COVID-19 patients who had been given remdesivir.

Noted researcher Dr. Pascal Sacré, in an article on the Global Research website with the intriguing title "COVID-19 – Remdesivir: License to Kill. Hydroxychloroquine: Prohibition to Cure," concluded: "Remdesivir can cause severe kidney failure (requiring dialysis, kidney transplant), liver failure, genetic mutation, heart problems up to cardiac arrest, among others. This is the truth." He also noted "Remdesivir's fight against Hydroxychloroquine (HCQ) is somewhat symbolic of the fight of medical journals, of corrupt institutions against field medicine, of the many general practitioners who are at the bedside."

A French publication said we "strongly believe that Veklury (remdesivir) is a harmful drug and that this evidence has been concealed by Gilead. We believe that the lobbying operation conducted in the media and certain public health authorities in order to discredit hydroxychloroquine, specifically in hospitals, was intended to make remdesivir the only solution in this situation."

Trump will have to be checked for some time for side effects from remdesivir.

Dr. Lee D. Merritt in an article in the Fall 2020 issue of the *Journal of the American Association of Physicians and Surgeons* unraveled the question of why Fauci has been so negative about HCQ: "Why is he so strongly promoting the $3,600 remdesivir and almost totally ignoring the $20 HCQ regimen, other than to say the latter is of 'unproven benefit'?" Are there conflicts of interest? She noted that Fauci is an integral part of a vaccine coalition, specifically the Global Vaccine Action Plan (GVAP), a collaboration of the Bill and Melinda Gates Foundation and Fauci's group. Fauci is also in the Leadership Council of the "Decade of Vaccines" Council. Large sums of money flow from the Gates Foundation to and around Fauci's projects.

Fauci's group also developed one of the currently tested vaccines in cooperation with the drug company Moderna, which has received nearly $500 million in federal funding for its work, and the NIH will likely receive significant money from the vaccine's use.

Even though Fauci is the highest paid federal employee, his incredibly high public exposure has resulted in other benefits. Ken McCarthy revealed in a *Veterans Today* June 2020 article, "Tony Fauci Is Corrupt to the Core!" that "The Albany Medical Center gave him half a million dollars for 'science innovation.' Now, it just happens that Albany Medical Center lives on NIH grants." This also was observed: "Fauci survives because he does what the deep state wants him to do. He's also a superb politician. And that's very important. He's got an M.D. degree. But the idea he's a physician is a joke. The idea that he's a scientist is a joke."

On the general issue of corruption in the pandemic, Dr. James Todaro said this in Fall 2020. "So over this past year the COVID-19 pandemic has really exposed or uncovered a tremendous amount of corruption and conflicts of interest that are in both the health sciences and medical fields." Because of "financial incentives we see so many of these health officials and organizations pushing a similar narrative—fear and panic—with the only way of getting back to a real normal (not the new normal) vaccine or Big Pharma therapeutic. I would say that the gatekeepers for the science overall are really the academic journals themselves. They are supposed to be the ones with the robust peer-reviewed processes to vet the science, to make sure there is valid and true science, with valid conclusions that are derived from the science. What we have seen is unprecedented corruption within those academic journals. In the past six months two of the top medical journals in the world, *The Lancet* and *The New England Journal of Medicine*, produced openly fraudulent studies that have benefited Big Pharma."

Part 4

—⁓ɷ⁓—

Developing a Personal Strategy to Stay Healthy

4.1 Expert views on lives that can be saved

The beginning of any personal strategy to stay healthy and survive the COVID pandemic is a deep appreciation for the undeniable truth that there are proven ways to save lives. This is the profound truth about the big pandemic blunder, meaning the failure of the public health system to support early home/outpatient COVID treatment as discussed in the previous parts of this book.

A number of statements by credible sources are presented to convince you of life-saving truths.

The White Paper on the website of America's Frontline Doctors by Dr. Simone Gold in the summer of 2020 concluded: "What we do know is that 70,000-100,000 excess American lives have been lost due to lack of access to HCQ."

On national television, Fox News in July 2020, Dr. Risch said, "Seventy-five to 100,000 lives will be saved" with use of the controversial medicine and that "we're basically fighting a propaganda war against the medical facts." Later in October 2020, after many more deaths, he said in *The Washington Examiner*: "Many or most of the 220,000 deaths in the United States to date could have been prevented by widespread HCQ use that the FDA blocked. It is the FDA that is responsible for these deaths, not the president." But Fauci is the power behind the throne, dictating FDA actions. What Risch said holds true now with a much higher number of deaths.

Dr. Brian Tyson has said that between 75 and 80 percent of the over 200,000 deaths thus far could have been prevented by using HCQ!

In November 2020, Dr. Peter McCollough said: "Public health historians will look back and call out a blunder. The lack of investment, execution of large-scale clinical trials, and implementation of available oral medications in a sequenced regimen, conceptualized by doctors in early April, was responsible for the greatest amount of human suffering and death in our nation's history. The avoidable loss of life is in the hundreds of thousands. The great gamble on the vaccine was a race in time in which 'warp speed' was simply not fast enough for those ill now and over the months to come before immunity closes out the crisis."

Also in November 2020, Dr. Zelenko said: "There is a cure for COVID-19 as well as effective prevention options. The Zelenko Protocol could have saved over 200,000 lives." Considering that this was when the national death figure was close to 280,000, this translates to about 70 percent of lives that could have been saved. But in his December 2020 published study "COVID-19 outpatients: early risk-stratified treatment with zinc plus low-dose hydroxychloroquine and azithromycin: a retrospective case series study" in the *International Journal of Antimicrobial Agents*, Zelenko found an 80 percent reduction in deaths among those receiving early home treatment with his protocol.

In November 2020, Sen. Ron Johnson, R-Wis., said thousands of people have died because doctors have ignored treating COVID-19 patients early with the use of alternative drugs, notably HCQ. "Thousands of people have died because we've ignored it. That's a question we're asking: why?" Johnson said, "There's a host of things we should have explored, we should be using, we should be letting doctors be doctors. And we should be celebrating their courage and their compassion rather than raking them over the coals and calling them names. ... this is ridiculous."

In December 2020, Dr. Ramin Oskoui, who appears often on Fox News, said that with HCQ use "probably over 100,000 deaths could've been easily avoided." How much over is the question. He added that because of the US rejection of hydroxychloroquine, "we've stressed our health care system, we've almost crashed our economy, and we've destroyed small business, and potentially, sadly, we may have really wounded ourselves from a military standpoint and a health care standpoint for years to come."

Also, in December 2020, Dr. Pierre Kory said: "The effective vaccines for which we have all been waiting are coming very soon, but not soon enough to save the tens of thousands who are projected to die before the widespread distribution of the vaccines can be completed. Right now, COVID-19 is a runaway train barreling down the tracks, and if you're on those tracks, ivermectin can help lift you out of harm's way."

In his December 2020 second senate hearing on early home/outpatient treatment, Senator Ron Johnson emphasized that probably hundreds of thousands of lives have been lost because of inattention to the use of the safe, low-cost HCQ and IVM generics for early home/outpatient treatment. At the same hearing, Dr. Rajter emphasized that "we cannot stand by and let hundreds of thousands of patients go untreated," with the clear inference that otherwise there would be hospitalizations and deaths. He emphasized that IVM destroys the COVID virus in forty-eight hours.

The most important point of the previously discussed data on the two sets of nations is that the data on the advantage of using HCQ (with a 70 percent reduction in deaths) imply saving about 200,000 U.S. lives in November 2020, when the total deaths were about 280,000. This savings figure of course will increase as the number of deaths, sadly, keeps increasing without wide use of home/outpatient use of HCQ or IVM, likely along with other medicines and supplements.

In sum, there is a clear, compelling, and medical basis for believing that a great many lives could have been saved and, in the future, could be saved through the use of the various medicines and protocols presented earlier. It is almost incomprehensible that we have a government and public health system that still is not doing everything feasible and proven to greatly reduce COVID deaths, in the range of 70 percent to 80 percent. It is morally repugnant and a disgrace. No wonder the terrific doctors active in the early home/outpatient treatment movement are filled with anger over what is not being used on a wide, national scale.

Knowing what you now know, consider this question. How can the omnipresent Fauci, who claims to follow science, ignore all the supporting evidence for preventing COVID deaths?

Again, if we had a truly objective, fair media, this number of saved lives, in the past and for the future, supported by what a number of doctors have said, that could be saved by using pillar one would make headlines. But the leftist mainstream media follows Fauci's lead.

The working paper titled "Why Is All COVID-19 News Bad News?" in November 2020, published by the National Bureau of Economic Research, reported an analysis of news stories about COVID-19 that appeared from January 1 through July 31. It found that 91 percent of the coverage by major US media outlets was "negative in tone." The rate was substantially lower in leading scientific journals (65 percent) and foreign sources (54 percent), but still very negative. Thank you, Fauci.

All the life-saving evidence is ignored by corrupt media and failed public health and government agencies. The leftist media would rather keep reporting rising cases, hospitalizations, and deaths. The aim is to push for more pounding contagion controls that keep going on despite the obvious reality that they have not worked after many months of use! And also, to keep up pressure to use vaccines.

Victor David Hanson, a leading conservative thinker, has introduced this apt description of the reality about leftist thinking stemming from the history with HCQ: "This Hydroxy Effect—hysterical disavowal of anything Trump has endorsed—is dangerous to the country at large."

Though the mainstream media has not done stories on all the lives that could have been saved by using early home/outpatient treatment, they have done countless articles blaming insufficient contagion controls for not preventing deaths. For most Americans, such a position seems ludicrous, considering so many months of disruptive and costly contagion controls, especially various types of lockdowns.

Senator Rand Paul had the right view of devastating lockdowns when he pointed out in December 2020 that there's no scientific evidence tyrannical lockdowns work: "You can take advice and you can give advice. But once you mandate it, it doesn't become advice. It becomes a form of tyranny."

Considering that so many medical professionals have documented the many negative health impacts of lockdowns, the failure to use life-saving early home/outpatient treatments is unfathomable, as is the media's lack of honest coverage of the entire COVID pandemic situation. This defines the big pandemic blunder, which was intentional and criminal.

4.2 How to get the best information and ignore and discount bad information and propaganda

This book is just the beginning of getting sound, reliable information to protect your life, whether or not you get a COVID vaccine. There has been far too much panic about the pandemic. The major reason for that is the strategy of the leftist media to weaponize negative data to maintain a crisis atmosphere enabling political powers to do what they want.

Then what do you do?

The first thing is to depend on information from "conservative" sources and avoid paying attention to COVID information from leftist, mainstream sources. In the former category are shows on Fox News, especially Tucker Carlson, Sean Hannity, and Laura Ingraham. There are a multitude of conservative websites, many of which have been identified in the previous parts of this book. Of particular note are websites that have published pandemic articles by this author; they include: WND.com, lifesitenews.com, globalresearch.ca, unz.com, opednews.com, nolanchart.com. Another important website is americasvoice.news, which airs the Steve Bannon war room show that has often given reliable information on the pandemic.

For data on the pandemic for the US and other nations is worldometers.info/coronavirus/.

Perhaps more importantly, ignore and discount COVID information that amounts to disinformation and propaganda on all the major leftist media, including the *Washington Post* and *New York Times*, as well as CNN and MSNBC. Stay away completely from social media for reliable information.

The most important habit to develop is to stop believing the endless statements and opinions spouted daily from the big mouth and loose lips of Fauci. You have to learn to not get suckered in by his soft voice and grandfatherly demeanor. Believe what a lot of smart medical professionals know, namely that Fauci does not deserve the unlimited and uncritical credibility the leftist media has given him for a long time.

Do not give him credit for following "the science." That line is just something Fauci has learned to use frequently as his way of justifying just about anything he is either promoting or criticizing. When others do something he supports, they are following the science. When others do something he disagrees with, they are not following the science. In other words, "the science" is up to Fauci to define as either good or bad. Of course, there really is objective science. Fauci chooses what science is legitimate or good science and what is bad from his biased perspective. He shows no respect for objective science. Of course, in any rapidly developing medical area there will be many sources of data, and they will differ from each other. But Fauci chooses only the data he likes and ignores all the rest.

Here is a good way to understand Fauci: Science means whatever a political tyrant wants it to mean.

On the subject of what scientific or medical data you can trust, this has become more difficult as journals that publish studies have increasingly come under criticism. There have been too many instances of articles that get past peer reviews only to be seen later as fraudulent or inaccurate and not worthy of being considered as good science. Too many journals and their editors seem to have a political agenda. Too many researchers have trouble getting articles accepted, because their data do not agree with a particular position. A good example are study data showing positive findings for HCQ.

If you pay close attention to exactly what Fauci says, you will notice over time that he rarely cites specific scientific or medical data. Part of his success as a propagandist is talking in generalities. This allows him to do what he always has done, namely change positions on important policies or actions. So, he can change from being against mask use to being for it. From being for school closings to being against them. Consider him a proverbial snake oil salesman. From comparing the COVID virus to a bad flu to proclaiming it a calamity. From saying you don't need to "change anything you're doing" to pushing strong contagion controls. From using models to predict deaths and telling reporters, "You can't really rely on models."

The use of some models by Fauci, notably the Imperial College model, to persuade President Trump to lock down the entire US economy had a devastating impact. At one point the fraudulent model predicted 2.2 million American deaths from the coronavirus pandemic. Many professionals called that model a sham and garbage. Did Fauci ever issue a public, heartfelt apology? No.

In November 2020, Senator Rand Paul, following Fauci's statement on ABC's *This Week* about prioritizing keeping schools open, stated that Fauci owes "every single parent and school-age child in America" an apology for prior statements.

In December 2020, Dr. Martin Kulldorff of Harvard said this about Fauci's views on pandemic management: "You need to know the infectious-disease epidemiology, and that is something that I have been studying for many decades, but it is not an area of expertise of Dr. Fauci. It is surprising to me that he makes statements on the epidemiology of the pandemic, which, to be honest, he has made a number of erroneous statements on this aspect. So that reduces the trust in public health again when people hear that and then realize that that was wrong." In other words, Fauci has never had a problem in limiting his public pronouncement on what he is truly expert on, which is not what he has done most of the time.

In January 2020, Fauci warned Trump that the nation was in real trouble, but the same month on television he told the public that the country did not have to worry and that the coronavirus was "not a major threat." Do you still want to trust what Fauci says?

In December 2020, Joy Pullmann in *The Federalist* summed things up nicely: "Fauci has shown himself, with the help of our anti-American media, highly effective at manipulating public perception. That's about all he's capable at, it seems."

One term that Fauci has used to justify his lack of support for HCQ is randomized controlled trial, discussed previously. To add more ammunition to disbelieving what Fauci says is his citing a lack of RCT for HCQ. First, any professional who deals with any aspect of drug testing and approval knows the vast literature that has shown over and over that RCTs are not the only sound way to get evidence that a drug is safe and effective. For sure, Fauci knew for decades that RCTs could never be used as the sole reason for denying government approval or support for a drug, especially a drug like HCQ that had long been used as an approved medicine for a number of diseases. Using HCQ for the COVID infection should have been allowed by the NIH and FDA. Fauci simply lied to the public when he invoked an absence of RCTs for HCQ. What incredible arrogance. He used an argument that countless professionals knew was hokum. But he went public with his argument because he knew it sounded sensible to uninformed, regular people. He used science to deceive and misinform the public. Just more reason as you try to use valid information to ignore what Fauci says.

Moreover, Fauci has ignored the federal law, discussed previously, that sanctions the use of Real World Evidence. As a fake scientist, Fauci has consistently failed to use so much available evidence given previously for using well-tested early home/outpatient treatments for COVID. Sensible Americans should always ask why Fauci has exhibited such corrupt behavior.

The more you believe what Fauci says, the more you will be risking your health and life. If you have come to fully appreciate all the negative aspects of Fauci, then watch and listen to him more as entertainment than a source of valid and useful information. There is value in understanding how Fauci is misleading and misdirecting Americans. In this way you will better appreciate that he is using disinformation and propaganda to advance his agenda, which is more political than medical. See Fauci as a corrupt person with incredible unchecked power. He is totally different than and inferior to the frontline doctors who have been taking so many risks in providing early home/outpatient COVID care. They are behaving against all the official government directives of the public health and regulatory systems.

Never forget that Fauci has used his power to block wide use of HCQ both as a prophylaxis and cure for COVID infection. The lack of guidance from the NIH for any home treatment also undercuts use of IVM by physicians, though Fauci has not spoken about it.

Even when you are exposed to information coming from the CDC and FDA, understand that they are like puppets who are being controlled by Fauci.

Dr. Jane Orient of the American Association of Physicians and Surgeons has made the great point that FDA has no legal authority to regulate the practice of medicine. Nevertheless, by its actions on HCQ, for example, it ends up doing exactly that.

One of the pioneers for early home treatment, Dr. George Fareed, in December 2020 emphasized this: "Sadly, many infected people and primary care doctors and doctors in ERs follow the NIH and Dr. Fauci stipulations with no effective treatments offered. We need to have the NIH/FDA/CDC formally acknowledge the importance of early treatment with moderately acting, safe antivirals so readily available. When (if ever) that happens, everything would improve dramatically."

Briefly, here are some points to remember if you hear about or read for yourself medical studies that conclude that HCQ or IVM is unsafe and ineffective.

Many such studies have used these drugs too late in the process of COVID infection. Mostly such studies have wrongly used what should be considered valid early treatment for hospitalized patients whose infection has progressed beyond the early virus replication stage. Although there have been many studies showing HCQ or IVM effective for hospitalized patients, the key is whether those patients were given the medicines early enough to be effective. But the majority of negative studies on HCQ or IVM gave the medicines too late to be effective.

In some other negative studies, the dosages of HCQ or IVM have been too high, or generally inconsistent with what positive studies have used successfully. Another shortcoming of many negative studies is that there was no use of zinc. Often negative studies include very small numbers of participants using the tested drug.

4.3 How to prepare for home/outpatient treatment

A basic decision is whether you want to obtain medicines and supplements that, as discussed in the previous section, have been found safe and effective for COVID prevention and cure.

Besides the information provided previously here, there are some very useful websites. Two of the best ones are the websites of America's Frontline Doctors and the American Association of Physicians and Surgeons. Both have details on protocols that have achieved respect by medical professionals.

Another very useful site is c19protocols.com. There are two main sections: one for early treatment and one for prevention. Each provides links to specific websites providing detailed information.

Yet another useful site that is updated frequently is covexit.com. It provides many videos covering both treatment and news. Of special value are videos featuring some successful frontline doctors using early home/outpatient COVID treatment. You must learn to use the feature at the bottom of the home page to progress to other pages.

A website particularly useful for getting information on prophylaxis is COVID19criticalcare.com. It tends to focus on the use of IVM rather than HCQ.

For getting links to published studies, go to c19study.com. It has sections on HCQ, IVM, supplements, as well as remdesivir.

Another useful website is medicineuncensored.com run by Dr. James Todaro, an early proponent of HCQ, that offers a broad range of useful information

Also to be used is the website of Dr. Zelenko (vladimirzelenko. com) that has much useful information. And the website rational-ground.com, which is also very useful.

4.4 New Medicines

While it is correct that the government has failed miserably in focusing on making the best use of repurposed generic drugs, such as HCQ and IVM, it has pursued new, mostly very expensive drugs. The US government has been especially negligent in acknowledging what a number of third world countries have done to effectively manage the coronavirus pandemic with low-cost generic drugs. This is a form of medical corruption.

For staying informed about new medicines, the TrialSiteNews.com website is very useful. And there will always be new drugs for treating COVID.

A good example is the work in the US to get a drug approved that is already being used in some other countries. That drug is favipiravir, a broad-spectrum antiviral that some medical professionals see as related to remdesivir. It is now a generic drug. It was tested, developed, and approved in Japan, with over 3,000 people safely using it. Unlike remdesivir, it is used as oral tablets and, therefore, can be used for early home/

outpatient COVID treatment. Note that this drug, like HCQ and IVM, may only offer benefits for early home/outpatient COVID treatment, and not for hospitalized patients with more advanced COVID infection. It has been reported that it has been successfully used in over thirty countries, including China and Russia, battling COVID-19.

Here is another newer treatment. Budesonide is an FDA-approved medication that decreases inflammation in the lungs. Inhaled budesonide is a safe, generic, inexpensive prescription medication. It is used by millions of people who suffer from asthma every day. Inhaled budesonide used with a nebulizer is believed to block the inflammatory chemicals released by the COVID virus and stop it from spreading.

Inhaled budesonide targets the lungs and does not affect your immune system or your body's ability to heal like systemic steroids do. It is likely that a doctor might also recommend using zinc and a common antibiotic.

Also getting attention is Regeneron's FDA-approved monoclonal antibody cocktail, given as an intravenous infusion. Federal funding supported its development. The Regeneron drug—which President Trump received during his hospitalization for COVID-19 in October—is not available to most people suffering from the virus. The cocktail antibody therapy uses two or more lab-engineered antibodies. Regeneron's cocktail includes a monoclonal antibody that targets the spike protein the virus uses to drill into healthy cells, and another antibody that targets a different part of the novel coronavirus. With the two, the goal is to trap and shut down viral replication. The treatment cost is at least $1,500. So far this product has been used for hospitalized patients, but it may also be available for outpatients.

The FDA has granted EUAs to remdesivir, convalescent plasma, a monoclonal antibody drug called bamlanivimab, and Regeneron's cocktail of monoclonal antibodies. As noted previously, the FDA previously granted and revoked EUA status for hydroxychloroquine, which many believe made it easier for the FDA to grant EUAs for other medicines and therapeutics.

4.5 How to find a doctor to get necessary medicines

As long as home/outpatient treatment is blocked by NIH guidelines denying approval for any such treatment, the vast majority of American doctors won't be using medicines like HCQ and IVM. That imposes a challenge on those people who want to use a protocol for either COVID prevention or early cure. There are three websites that offer assistance in finding a doctor who can help you get a safe and proven protocol.

The website c19protocols.com has a section "physicians/facilities offering early treatment." There are many links that are very useful in finding doctors to consider. One of the best links is to the American Association of Physicians and Surgeons (aapsonline.org) that you can access separately. This group has an extensive listing of doctors in specific locations across the nation. It also has a free, extremely useful document titled "A Guide to Home-Based COVID Treatment." This is regularly updated.

Another good website is americasfrontlinedoctors.com. It offers a detailed section on obtaining HCQ. Users can check what their state situation is for obtaining HCQ. Another section helps users find a doctor and prescription through use of telemedicine.

4.6 What to think about if needing hospitalization

Anyone who is hospitalized with COVID infection—likely meaning that a combination of symptoms and test results has caused a physician to determine the need for hospitalization—should seriously inquire what medicines and protocols are available.

With priority given these days in nearly all hospitals of using patient-centered care, patients and their advocates have every right to inquire about whether the newest and best medicines and protocols are being offered and used, and what data are available on how successful the hospital has been in treating COVID patients and avoiding longer term problems. There clearly have been great advances in hospital treatment for COVID, with much better results for preventing deaths. But still, there is no substitute for patients and their family advocating for themselves to get the best available treatment.

4.7 Dealing with pandemic developments

The biggest pandemic development hitting the public is the availability of COVID vaccines. Still, there are issues and uncertainties that are likely to cause many Americans to resist taking a vaccine. Whether there is long-term immunity, for example, remains an issue. And it may take a long time for clear evidence that there is still no significant spreading of the COVID disease, because of herd immunity.

In December 2020, Fauci said this with regard to COVID vaccines: "We have the gold standard of a regulatory approach with the FDA." What few people seem to understand is that the vaulted randomized controlled trials so often invoked by Fauci have not been used by the government to prove the safety and effectiveness of COVID vaccines.

It should also be noted that in July 2020, Fauci clearly said that the coronavirus would never be eradicated, despite contagion controls and use of vaccines. At best, he said only control of the virus was possible. This view does not promote public optimism about taking a vaccine.

On the official FDA website is a presentation titled "Safety Surveillance of COVID-19 Vaccines," dated October 22, 2020, there was a list of twenty-two possible adverse outcomes. It is a breathtaking list of various diseases, including stroke, acute myocardial infarction, anaphylaxis, autoimmune disease, death, arthritis and arthralgia/joint pain, for example.

In late 2020, a controversy developed concerning the inclusion of HIV material in some vaccines, including one developed in Australia that was removed from use because of false positive tests for HIV. In October 2020, an article in *The New York Post* had the headline "Some COVID-19 vaccines could increase risk of HIV, researchers warn." This was noted: "Some coronavirus vaccine candidates currently under development could increase susceptibility to HIV, a group of researchers has warned. A modified virus being used in four COVID-19 vaccine contenders—called adenovirus 5 (Ad5)—has been shown to increase transmission of the AIDS virus in the past, the researchers wrote in a 'cautionary tale' published on October 19, 2020 in *The Lancet* medical journal."

A *Forbes* magazine article on the same issue titled "Researchers Warn Some COVID-19 Vaccines Could Increase Risk Of HIV Infection" included this: "Exactly how the vaccine increased the risks of HIV transmission is unknown, but a conference convened by the National Institutes of Health recommended against further use of Ad5 as a vector in HIV vaccines (Dr. Anthony Fauci was lead author of the [2014] paper outlining this position.).”

A December 2020 research paper titled “The Potential for SARS-CoV-2 to Evade Both Natural and Vaccine-induced Immunity” said: “It also seems likely that reinfection with a variant strain of SARS-CoV-2 may occur among people who recover from COVID-19, and that vaccines with the ability to generate antibodies against multiple variant forms of the spike protein will be necessary to protect against variant forms of SARS-CoV-2 that are already circulating in the human population.” In other words, reinfection is a real possibility, even after getting a vaccine.

Here is another facet to the issue of vaccine safety that probably few people are aware of. Congress took action in April 2020 that stipulates that companies “cannot be sued for money damages in court” over injuries caused by medical countermeasures for COVID-19. Such countermeasures include vaccines, therapeutics, and respiratory devices. This action bars anyone who feels they were harmed by a vaccine for the coronavirus from using the National Vaccine Injury Compensation Program. In September 2020, the HHS Secretary made it very clear: “Any treatment or vaccine for purposes of a national emergency pandemic like this actually comes with liability protection,” Azar explained. “Both the product as well as those who administer it or provide it.”

Many other countries have also given COVID vaccine makers protection. But a December 2020 article in *The Hill* noted that European Union officials “have refused to offer any blanket liability protection to promising vaccine candidates, instead choosing to haggle with each individual vaccine maker over liability limits terms. Those negotiations have delayed vaccine contract negotiations for months, leaving the average European at the back of the vaccine queue." Meaning that orders for vaccines were held up.

Staying abreast of new treatments for home/outpatient use will remain a challenge. Though there is a constant flow of information from local public health agencies and the media, as discussed earlier, one needs a critical-thinking and skeptical mindset to not fall victim of disinformation and outright propaganda. There really has been a big pandemic blunder that should not be forgotten or dismissed. That the national health care, public health, regulatory, and political systems successfully kept early home/outpatient COVID treatment out of the limelight and out of easy use by Americans has been a national tragedy and disgrace.

For the foreseeable future there will be daily news across all media on the coronavirus disease and the ways to manage it. Public officials from all levels of government will continue to deliver opinions, data, and directives. Mostly, they will focus on the many forms of contagion controls, such as masks and lockdowns, and using vaccines. As this book has shown, public officials and people like Fauci no longer deserve much public trust. The burden on you is to use the information sources given credence in this book to stay healthy.

As to the choice between using one of the protocols for early COVID treatment versus vaccination, here is what Ivette C. Lozano, MD said in December 2020: "I have personally treated 950+ Covid 19 patients in my office successfully with Hydroxychloroquine, Zithromax & Zinc. The reluctance of physicians to treat patients with Hydroxychloroquine and the refusal of hospitals to administer

Hydroxychloroquine is in my opinion inhumane. The withholding of medical care in no way warrants mass vaccination of the public with a vaccine that has been rushed to market with limited safety studies for a disease that remains 99% survivable. I plead with you to administer Hydroxychloroquine to your patients and save their lives."

As 2020 turned into 2021 the leftist news storm ignored three critically important revelations. Senator Marco Rubio had the guts to say publicly that "Fauci lied about coronavirus to manipulate our behavior." He criticized placing blind faith in unelected celebrity scientists. Prompting this was that Fauci had admitted in an interview with the New York Times that he had intentionally lied about the percent of Americans needing covid vaccination to reach herd immunity. Earlier he said that 60 to 70 percent would work. Then 90 percent. Fauci used public polls, not science, to shape what he told the public.

Not everyone has swallowed the propaganda about Fauci. Note that Nobel Prize winner Kary Mullis said "Tony Fauci does not mind going on television in front of the people, face out, and lie directly into the camera."

Fauci also revealed in a Newsweek interview that covid vaccines were not proven to stop covid infection and transmission even if they worked to stop serious health impacts. Contagion controls, like masks and lockdowns, would continue. World Health Organization's chief scientist agreed.

The esteemed Dr. Peter McCollough made this critical observation in December 2020: "Because the Pfizer-BioNTech and Moderna clinical trials were analyzed prematurely after 2 of the planned 24 months of observation, we simply cannot know at this time if the vaccination will provide durable protection." And Gerald Williams smartly observed: "Of course if only there wasn't suppression of early HCQ/Zn and Ivermectin based treatment protocols, we wouldn't have needed a vaccine and the country would have been open months ago."

Importantly, several investigations revealed that 40 percent of supposedly covid deaths resulted from other things, such as gunshot wounds, automobile and motorcycle accidents, and influenza. Dying with covid is not the same as dying because of covid infection. Also, covid hospitalization data were fear mongering. Financial incentives pushed hospitals, doctors and public health agencies to over diagnose.

An impressive report "Lockdowns Do Not Control the Coronavirus: The Evidence" by the American Institute for Economic Research, in December 2020 came to these important conclusions.

"The use of universal lockdowns in the event of the appearance of a new pathogen has no precedent. It has been a science experiment in real time, with most of the human population used as lab rats. The costs are legion. The question is whether lockdowns worked to control the virus in a way that is scientifically verifiable. The answer is no and for a variety of reasons: bad data, no correlations, no causal demonstration, anomalous exceptions, and so on. There is no relationship between lockdowns (or whatever else people want to call them to mask their true nature) and virus control.... In a saner world, the burden of proof really should belong to the lockdowners, since it is they who overthrew 100 years of public-health wisdom and replaced it with an untested, top-down imposition on freedom and human rights.... The anti-lockdown studies ...are evidence-based, robust, and thorough, grappling with the data we have (with all its flaws) and looking at the results in light of controls on the population."

This is what the evidence shows: Untrustworthy data maintains public fear that justifies continued virus controls used by political forces with a thirst for power over citizens.

Here is final advice for readers of this book:

Never forget the many thousands of American lives that could have been saved, but medicines that work early to cure the COVID disease were intentionally blocked and not widely used.

Remember the history of medicine lesson: Always treat a disease as early as possible.

Remember that the collusion between Fauci and the leftist media to withhold effective early treatment has ruined the lives of so many and killed many Americans. A terrible debacle of historic significance.

CPSIA information can be obtained
at www.ICGtesting.com
Printed in the USA
BVHW031734090321
602112BV00008B/681